F

D1716136

# Intervention Activities for At-Risk Youth

# Intervention Activities for At-Risk Youth

by Norma J. Stumbo

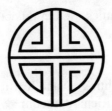

Venture Publishing, Inc.
State College, Pennsylvania

Production Manager: Richard Yocum
Design, Layout, Graphics, and Manuscript Editing: Diane K. Bierly
Additional Editing: Deborah L. McRann and Richard Yocum
Cover Design and Illustration: Diane K. Bierly

Library of Congress Catalogue Card Number 99-64586
ISBN 1-892132-07-9

# Contents

*Contents*

# Acknowledgments

Mr. Bill Gillis, Chief Executive Officer, Dr. Robert Lusk, Director of Clinical Services, and Ms. Karen Rousey, Director of Residential Treatment Center, at The Baby Fold in Normal, Illinois, have been tremendous supporters of the Illinois State University therapeutic recreation students who worked diligently on activities in this manual. They are to be thanked for their insights, patience, and commitment to providing the best services possible. The entire staff at The Baby Fold, a Normal, Illinois, residential treatment facility for at-risk youth, has embraced the concept of intervention programming through recreation activities and have supported both the students and activities manual project.

Appreciation also is extended to the faculty of the Recreation and Park Administration Program at Illinois State University, especially to the former and current therapeutic recreation faculty, Drs. Patricia B. Malik and Cynthia J. Wachter. Collegial support is always needed for a project of this size. Sandra Larson, an ISU therapeutic recreation master's degree alumna, wrote the final versions of the second and third chapters and is to be acknowledged for staying when the staying got tough. Two former Illinois State University therapeutic recreation students, Theresa Connolly and Amy Grabowski, worked on drafts of the first three chapters and edited many of the activities. Master's degree alumnae, Mary Hess and Amanda McGowen, also helped to edit many of the activities and supervised students as they completed fieldwork at The Baby Fold. It's an absolute delight to have such talented and dedicated students with whom to work. Michelle Schuline, Office of Undergraduate Studies at Illinois State University, is thanked for her patience and computer skills in finalizing the text to go to the publisher.

Of course, some of the most significant contributions came from the former undergraduate therapeutic recreation students who created the activities found in this manual. Virtually all of these activities have been used with at-risk youth and were created to address specific needs of at-risk youth. The students displayed an enormous amount of creative energy and knowledge of intervention programming to design the activities in this manual. Their contributions to this manual are monumental as I suspect their contributions to the profession will be.

The contributors are listed alphabetically below:

Kristen Boys
Connie Campbell
Theresa M. Connolly
Amy Conron
Kate Czerwinski
Julie Harvey
Jessica Kamm
Lisa Koerner
Sandra Larson
Jennifer Matkowich
Amanda L. McGowen
Susan Osborn
Renee Raczkowski
Monika Ressel
Courtney Stauffer
Craig W. Strohbeck
Lazheta Thomas

# Preface

*Intervention Activities for At-Risk Youth* represents a unique, professional, symbiotic relationship between The Baby Fold and the Recreation and Park Administration program at Illinois State University. The Baby Fold wanted intervention recreation activities delivered to their children, but did not have adequate resources to employ a full-time therapeutic recreation specialist. A connection was made with the therapeutic recreation faculty at Illinois State, and a specially designed fieldwork experience was created at The Baby Fold for therapeutic recreation undergraduate students. Students who completed the fieldwork designed, implemented, and evaluated intervention activities for the youth at the residential treatment facility. Students documented these successful activities and the best of the activities were collected and edited into *Intervention Activities for At-Risk Youth.* In turn, The Baby Fold receives all royalties from the sale of the activities manual, for the sole purpose of employing a therapeutic recreation specialist.

The benefits from this unique relationship have had an effect on a number of parties. The Illinois State students received valuable working experience and are able to see their efforts in print. The Baby Fold will enjoy the professional contributions of a therapeutic recreation specialist. Readers will have an excellent resource of tried and tested activities that work with at-risk youth. And, of course, the youth themselves—both at The Baby Fold and at other service facilities throughout the country—will benefit from being the recipients of intervention activities that will help minimize their "at-riskness."

The chapters and activity sections are intended both for those facilities that do and do not employ professional therapeutic recreation staff. The activities and goals are written in a format that a variety of staff, from volunteers to childcare workers to activity staff to professional therapeutic recreation specialists, can utilize in implementing intervention activities for at-risk youth.

The first three chapters provide a foundation for intervention activities—that is, activities that are implemented to bring about a positive change in the youths' behavior. The first introductory chapter outlines the needs of at-risk youth and a rationale for the activity sections that follow. The second chapter provides a brief overview of how to design, implement, and evaluate intervention activities, while the third provides a variety of activity resources.

The activities are divided into six sections:

- anger control and stress management (13 activities);
- positive physical and mental health (31 activities);
- cooperation, communication, and listening (26 activities);
- problem-solving, decision-making, and planning skills (17 activities);
- leisure awareness and leisure resources (49 activities); and
- friendship and social skills (33 activities).

These six areas were selected very specifically to address the needs of at-risk youth. In all, these 169 activities are meant to help professionals serving at-risk youth establish active treatment goals for the youth and move them toward more positive behaviors.

## Chapter One

# At-Risk Youth

The term *at-risk youth* is both a helpful and trouble-some one. It is helpful in that it brings attention to a group of individuals who are likely to need intervention to avert potentially dangerous circumstances. It is troublesome in that the same group of individuals is quite diverse, to the point of defying a solid and concrete classification system. So on one hand, as we try to classify them, for example for the purpose of providing services, their very diversity makes it difficult to do so.

McWhirter, McWhirter, McWhirter, and McWhirter (1995) highlight three important dimensions to the term *at risk:* "(a) the future time dimensions inherent in the term, (b) at risk as a continuum rather than a dichotomy, and (c) interactions between treatment and prevention" (p. 567). Resnick and Burt (1996) agreed that the term *at risk* implied some future orientation. They defined risk as:

> The presence of negative antecedent conditions (risk antecedents), which create vulnerabilities, combined with the presence of specific early negative behavior or experiences (risk markers) that are likely to lead, in time, to problem behavior that will have more serious long-term health consequences (health outcomes). (p. 174)

While their definition will be discussed more fully later, it is important to note that, by some individuals, *at risk* is used in a predictive fashion, that is, that future negative behaviors or consequences are anticipated in absence of specific intervention.

## At-Risk Continuum

McWhirter et al. (1993, 1995) also discussed the concept of a continuum of being at risk. The five components of their continuum include (a) minimal risk, (b) remote risk, (c) high risk, (d) imminent risk, and (e) participation in at-risk behaviors. They emphasized that there is no such thing as "no risk," because every individual can fall prey to destructive patterns, regardless of risk potential:

- *Minimal risk:*
  - are members of families of high socio-economic status;
  - have few psychosocial stressors;
  - attend good schools; and
  - have loving, caring relationships with families and friends.
- *Remote risk:*
  - families of low socioeconomic status;
  - membership in minority ethnic group;
  - less than positive family, school, and social interactions;
  - increased psychosocial stressors (divorce or death in immediate family); and
  - loss of family income.
- *High risk:*
  - individual's personal negative attitudes and emotions, such as depression, anxiety, aggression, hopelessness;
  - social skills deficits and poor coping behaviors; and
  - internalization of personal problems.

- *Imminent risk:*
    - gateway behaviors—mildly or moderately distressing activities;
    - self-destructive behaviors;
    - deviant behaviors, such as aggression toward other children and authority (e.g., gateway to juvenile delinquency); and
    - advances from cigarettes to alcohol to marijuana to harder drugs.
- *At-risk activity:*
    - have passed beyond risk because they have already exhibited maladaptive behavior;
    - if already involved in one activity, become at risk for other behaviors; and
    - at-risk behavior likely to continue into adulthood.

Another continuum mentioned by McWhirter et al. (1993, 1995) is whether services are provided in the preventative mode or the remedial mode. Not surprisingly, the preventative mode looks at youth in the minimal, remote, high-risk, and perhaps, imminent-risk categories. Remedial programs (such as juvenile detention) are more likely offered to individuals who are classified as having participated in risk activity (such as criminal behavior). The full spectrum of services (preventative to remedial) are important to serving the full range of at-risk categories (minimal to risk behavior).

# Resnick and Burt's Adolescent Risk Model

Resnick and Burt (1996) presented a different model that also, in its own way, presents a continuum of being at risk. Their model, titled the Adolescent Risk Model, provides a conceptual framework for understanding the variability of at-risk characteristics and implications of behavior. "From an ecological perspective, youth at risk are more likely to come from environments that heighten their vulnerability—communities with a dearth of social resources, high levels of stress, and inadequate institutional support" (p. 174). As such, the authors believed that there are four major categories of variables that "predict" at riskness: (a) antecedents, (b) markers, (c) behavior, and (d) outcomes.

Antecedents are those conditions that predict significant negative outcomes for youth (for example, poverty, neighborhood environment, family dysfunction, and lack of parental involvement and/or support). Markers are behaviors or conditions that signal impending dysfunction (such as poor school performance, being placed out of the home). Problem behaviors are those that have negative consequences for the individual or community in which he or she lives. Problem behaviors include early initiation of sexual behavior, running away, school truancy or absenteeism, and early use of tobacco and drugs. Outcomes include the results of the problem behaviors. Typical outcomes include teenage pregnancy and parenthood, homelessness, prostitution, sexually transmitted diseases, dropping out of school, committing crimes, imprisonment, morbidity, and mortality (Resnick and Burt, 1996).

By including community, family, and individual factors, the Adolescent Risk Model (Resnick and Burt, 1996), provides a multivariate approach to understanding the complex interactions that present a youth at risk. This model has implications for understanding at-risk youth as well as designing and providing services for them. More information on the latter point will be discussed later in this chapter.

# Kelley's Neocognitive Learning Theory

Another perspective on at-risk youth comes from Kelley (1993). In his paper on understanding the relationship between cognition, emotion, and delinquent behavior, Kelley presented an interesting set of assumptions that may impact how services are designed and implemented for at-risk youth. The first assumption is that "every child begins life with a natural, inborn capacity for healthy psychological functioning. That is, at birth, children do not have the mind-set which points them toward delinquency, drug use, or other forms of deviant behavior" (p. 440). Kelley argued that children are born with the capacity of healthy functioning, including common sense, a desire to learn, motivation for prosocial lifestyles, unconditional and positive self-worth, desire to learn, and a sense of mastery in learning about the environment. Kelley believed further that high self-esteem is inherent in each individual and is not derived originally from external stimuli.

The second major assumption of the neocognitive learning theory is that delinquent and dysfunctional behaviors are a result of external forces. A negative frame of reference is learned through unconditioned learning (based on personal insight and intuition) and conditioned learning (based on fear and insecurity when external forces do not agree with internal feelings). This means that external feedback that presents negative information about the child ("You're so stupid!"), creates a sense of insecurity and questioning that alienates the child from his or her original feelings of high self-worth.

The third major assumption, according to Kelley (1993), is that a child's original feelings of adequacy and healthy self-image can be reconstructed regardless of prior history and feelings of insecurity. That is, behavior that can be learned, can be relearned in a different fashion. Old feelings of adequacy and self-worth that were once part of a person's makeup can be rekindled through specific interventions and treatments. This provides great hope for individuals serving youth who are at risk.

# Vulnerability Versus Resiliency

The review of these three models or theories (cf., Kelley, 1993; McWhirter et al., 1993, 1995; Resnick and Burt, 1996) begs the question: Why do some youth exhibit at-risk behaviors and others, in the same environment and under the same conditions, do not? What makes some individuals resilient and some individuals vulnerable? While there likely is no single answer to these questions, one potential key is how the individual internally negotiates those environments and conditions. Similar to the point made by Kelley (1993), each person is born as a psychologically healthy, problem-solving, thinking individual. What that person learns while negotiating with external demands and internal interpretations, will affect how that individual views the world and views himself or herself.

For the most part, youth who are considered at risk for potentially negative future life events are those who are vulnerable to their surrounding conditions. Their negotiations with their world have left them with negative interpretations of their own skills, competence, and self-definition. In many ways, vulnerable individuals enter a downward spiral of a self-fulfilling prophecy that believes external others are in control and their own efforts have no or little effect.

McWhirter et al. (1993) used the term *resilient* to refer to individuals who could problem solve, make healthy decisions, and survive even under the most dire conditions. Resilient individuals are those who exhibit competence, autonomy, and effective strategies to cope; those who experience adverse developmental conditions and are still able to live productive, normal lives (McWhirter et al., 1993, p. 85). Common characteristics of resilient youth include:

- have an active approach to life's problems, able to negotiate emotionally hazardous experiences;
- perceive pain, frustration, and other distressing experiences constructively;
- are able to gain positive attention from others;
- possess strong faith that maintains a vision of a positive and meaningful life; and
- displays competence in social, school, and cognitive areas.

Youth who are resilient are seen as low risk. Characteristics which help to discriminate between low-risk and high-risk youth, as identified by McWhirter et al., (1993), include:

- critical school competencies, such as basic academic skills and academic survival skills;
- concept of self and self-esteem, which includes such concepts as ability to influence change;
- social and interpersonal skills, such as communication with others and perspective taking;
- ability to cope productively with anxiety and stress; and
- center of control, such as taking personal responsibility and having a life purpose.

High-risk or vulnerable youth often are deficient in one or more of these areas. The lack of these skills often is closely related to dependency, aggressive behavior, or the inability to cope with life stressors.

Youth who are deficient in *critical school competencies* lack basic reasoning, writing, and arithmetic skills. Youth who lack these skills tend to underachieve and often demonstrate behavior patterns of

*Intervention Activities for At-Risk Youth*

anger and defiance or apathy and withdrawal (McWhirter et al., 1993). In addition to this lack of basic skills, these high-risk youth also lack classroom survival skills including (a) attending to task; (b) following directions; (c) raising one's hand to ask or answer questions; and (d) writing legibly.

These high-risk youth, who may be underachievers academically, may engage in antisocial, deviant behaviors as a method of increasing *self-esteem,* due to their lack of experience with success. High-risk youth often have a distorted self-concept which affects their self-esteem. Self-concept is the way in which people perceive themselves in a variety of areas—academically, physically, socially. Self-esteem is the way in which an individual evaluates these self-concept perceptions. Because high-risk youth have a distorted self-concept, McWhirter et al. (1993) stated that these youth then perceive things negatively and lower their own expectations for success.

In addition to academic underachievement and a negative self-concept, high-risk youth also tend to be deficient in *social, communication, coping, and self-control skills.* High-risk youth often lack the core skills required for satisfying social relationships, which according to McWhirter et al., (1993) include:

- developing and maintaining friends;
- sharing laughter and jokes with peers;
- knowing how to join group activity;
- skillfully ending a conversation; and
- interacting with a variety of peers and others.

The ability to *cope effectively with anxiety and stress* is another skill that differentiates low-risk youth. Resilient youth often use patterns of humor and altruism, or tend to focus attention elsewhere when coping with stressors. High-risk youth often are observed utilizing patterns of compulsive acting out, withdrawal, denial, anxiety, and depression when coping with stressors (McWhirter et al., 1993).

These evasive methods of coping utilized by high-risk youth are related closely to their *inability to demonstrate self-control.* McWhirter et al. (1993) stated that high-risk youth fail to consider consequences, are unwilling to delay gratification, and operate on an external locus (center) of control. High-risk youth have difficulty with setting constructive and attainable goals and feel that events in their lives

and even their own behaviors are controlled by forces outside of themselves. High-risk youth feel they have no power to shape their own lives (McWhirter et al., 1993).

# Skills Needed by At-Risk Youth

The previously stated information points to the fact that often at-risk youth need specific intervention in developing necessary skills. These skills typically fall into the categories of:

- anger control and stress management;
- positive physical and mental health;
- cooperation, communication, and listening skills;
- problem-solving, decision-making, and planning skills;
- leisure awareness and leisure resources; and
- friendship and social skills.

While these skills can be taught in a variety of ways, often youth learn more, and have more fun while learning, if the skills are taught through active involvement. These six categories are used to organize intervention activities within this manual.

Here are some typical goals for at-risk youth in each of these categories:

- *Anger control and stress management:*
  - to improve ability to control anger outbursts,
  - to express anger in appropriate ways,
  - to identify situations that the child finds stressful, and
  - to identify methods to manage and reduce stress;
- *Positive physical and mental health:*
  - to learn ways to improve physical health,
  - to improve physical fitness through exercise,
  - to improve personal outlook on the future, and
  - to appreciate self and others;
- *Cooperation, communication, and listening skills:*
  - to cooperate with peers on a mutual task,
  - to communicate needs assertively,

4

- to listen to peers without interruption, and
- to increase knowledge of nonverbal body language;
- *Problem-solving, decision-making, and planning skills:*
  - to identify options for solution to problem,
  - to select best options for problem solution from among many,
  - to make decision regarding daily activities, and
  - to plan for a recreation out-trip;
- *Leisure awareness and leisure resources:*
  - to identify importance of leisure in one's daily life,
  - to increase awareness of community resources for involvement,
  - to identify agency resources to do on one's own, and
  - to identify benefits from participating in recreation activities;
- *Friendship and social skills:*
  - to improve conversational skills with peers and others,
  - to improve manners in public settings,
  - to identify important characteristics of friends, and
  - to identify personal strengths and weaknesses as a friend.

The activities in this manual are designed around these six areas, and the goals stated here are typical of those found in the activity plans that follow. The next chapter overviews how to design intervention activities and can help the reader select those activities that best meet the needs of the children and youth in a particular setting. The next chapter not only provides a rationale for providing intervention activities for at-risk youth, but also shows the childcare professional how to design activities if additional exercises are needed.

# Summary

Most authors agree that a continuum of "at riskness" exists. While every youth has potential, those who are found in certain environments or have certain characteristics are more likely to develop maladaptive behaviors that will have lifelong effects. Those who are most vulnerable are most at risk. Vulnerable children often are deficient in school skills, have low self-esteem, minimal social skills, ineffective coping and stress management skills, and have an external (versus internal) locus of control. The 168 intervention activities in this manual are in six categories to address these needs of the most vulnerable and at-risk youth.

# References

Kelley, T. M. (1993). Neocognitive learning theory: Implications for prevention and early intervention strategies with at-risk youth. *Adolescence, 28*(110), 439–460.

McWhirter, J. J., McWhirter, B. T., McWhirter, A. M., & McWhirter, E. H. (1993). *At-risk youth: A comprehensive response.* Pacific Grove, CA: Brooks/Cole Publishing Company.

McWhirter, J. J., McWhirter, B. T., McWhirter, A. M., & McWhirter, E. H. (1995). Youth at risk: Another point of view. *Journal of Counseling & Development, 73,* 567–569.

Resnick, G., & Burt, M. R. (1996). Youth at risk: Definitions and implications for service delivery. *American Journal of Orthopsychiatry, 66*(2), 172–183.

## Chapter Two

# Designing Intervention Programs for At-Risk Youth

## by Sandra Larson

There are two basic types of activity programming. For the purpose of this chapter, the terms *recreation programming* and *intervention programming* will be used. Recreation programming refers to activities that are structured and designed to provide an opportunity for participants to engage in recreation activities for the purpose of an enjoyable experience. Intervention programming is the process of choosing or designing activities that are aimed at producing a specific behavior change in the child. Although the two categories of programming are very different, they are in fact complementary as well. Figure 1 illustrates the distinctions between the two categories more clearly.

General recreation activities have the potential to add significantly to a child's development. Let's examine some benefits of recreation programming. Recreation programs:

- are flexible;
- can be targeted to meet the needs of the individual child;
- are easily modified to fit a specific purpose; and

- can offer a change of pace from more traditional treatment.

Based on this information, it is important to understand that recreation activities have great potential to contribute to a child's treatment goals and overall ability to function successfully in the community if the activities have been designed with prior, intentional planning. If the activities provided to the child are to be complementary to other forms of treatment, they can be designed to address very specific needs of the children and are, therefore, intervention in nature. For example, if a child has great difficulty interacting appropriately with his or her peers, activities can be designed in a very structured sequence that helps the child learn the appropriate interaction skills. Specifically, a child may first be taught to interact cooperatively with one child, then more than one child, and then taught the positive competitive skills necessary for team sport participation. It is important to note that in order to be a successful intervention programmer, there are four basic principles to which one must adhere when designing intervention-based

---

**Figure 1: Distinctions Between Intervention and Recreation Activities**

| Intervention Activities | Recreation Activities |
|---|---|
| *Purpose:* To change a specific behavior | *Purpose:* To provide opportunity for enjoyment |
| *Goals:* Outcome-oriented and measurable | *Goals:* Less well-defined and global |
| *Structure:* Higher degree of structure | *Structure:* Lesser degree of structure (usually) |
| *Evaluation:* Focus is on child's outcome | *Evaluation:* Focus is on child's enjoyment |
| *Outcomes:* Specific behavior change | *Outcomes:* Enjoyment, fun, exposure to activities |

programs for at-risk youth. These four principles are as follows:

1. Role modeling appropriate behavior is not enough to create a change. Structured skill-building activities, complete with goals, objectives, and projected outcomes need to be in place.
2. Only those children who need the program should be placed in the program.
3. Only those activities that are most likely to result in changed behavior should be used in the intervention program as part of the treatment.
4. The activity chosen should be looked at in detail before, during, and after implementation to determine how well the activity is assisting the child in creating a change.

Based on the four principles, this chapter will look at the essential components of designing intervention programs for at-risk youth. Specifically, sequential steps to designing intervention programs will be discussed. These steps include:

- development of the program's statement of purpose,
- program goals,
- child goals and objectives,
- child assessment,
- activity analysis and modification, and
- activity evaluation.

Again, intervention programming is crucial in creating a positive behavioral change in at-risk youth. The purpose of this chapter is to assist childcare workers, who work with at-risk youth, to create quality intervention programs and activities.

# Principle #1

*Role modeling appropriate behavior is not enough to create a change; structured skill-building activities, complete with goals, objectives, and projected outcomes need to be in place.*

According to Peterson and Gunn (1984), the term *specific program* is defined as "a designated set of activities and interventions designed to meet the pre-determined set of objectives for a specific group of clients" (p. 57). Individual activities that are grouped into specific programs are selected based on the needs of the children and youth. For example, through the literature, we found six areas in which most at-risk youth are deficient. We selected these six areas to develop activities, based on the identified needs of the children and youth. These individual activities could be designed into an overall program that moves children and youth to more positive behaviors. (An individual activity is likely to have minimal impact on its own; several activities in a cohesive series [a program] are usually more likely to achieve the intended results.)

When providing intervention-oriented activities for at-risk youth, the leader must strategically and appropriately place the selected activities into a specific program. For example, a specific program that would be beneficial for almost all at-risk youth is Social Interaction Skills. Included in the specific program is a statement of purpose, program goals, child goals, and child objectives.

## Statement of Purpose

The statement of purpose is "a concise, one-sentence explanation of the program's focus" (Peterson and Gunn, 1984, p. 91). The statement of purpose also must align with an agency's mission and philosophy, as well as the scope of the agency's service. In other words, when developing a specific program statement of purpose, be sure to refer to the agency's statement of purpose to ensure that the two complement each other. An example of a specific statement of purpose is as follows:

> *Specific Program:* Social Interaction Skills
> *Statement of Purpose:* To provide activities that assist in the improvement, maintenance, and utilization of appropriate social interaction skills that can be used in a variety of settings and situations.

Notice that the purpose statement does not attempt to provide information regarding how the program will be delivered or for whom the program is created (Peterson and Gunn, 1984, p. 91). The sole responsibility of the specific program's statement of purpose is to provide a "statement of intent" (Peterson and Gunn, 1984, p. 91). However, the statement of purpose provides the childcare worker with a solid foundation regarding program goals, which is the next step in developing an intervention-based program.

## Program Goals

Program goals can be viewed as general outcome statements that provide a framework for the content of the specific program. The main function of a specific program goal is to provide the leader with a "further explanation or definition of the program's purpose" (Peterson and Gunn, 1984, p. 93). To achieve this, creating more than one specific program goal will be necessary. Even though their needs tend to cluster (for example, social skills), children often have multiple needs in one area (for example, interacting with peers, manners, conversational skills, and hygiene are all social interaction skills). Each area can be represented by a goal statement.

The following are some examples of specific program goals that correlate with the statement of purpose noted in the Social Interaction Skills example:

> *Specific Program:* Social Interaction Skills
> *Statement of Purpose:* To provide activities that assist in the improvement, maintenance, and utilization of appropriate social interaction skills that can be used in a variety of settings and situations.
> *Specific Program Goals:*
> 1. To teach the child to engage in conversation with peers, adults, and authority figures.
> 2. To teach the child methods of communicating effectively specific needs, wants, and requests for assistance.
> 3. To instruct the child in engaging appropriately in dual and small group interactions.
> 4. To educate the child in the development of appropriate manners when with peers and authority figures in classroom, home, and community settings.
> 5. To train the child to identify and utilize appropriate expression of emotions.

Programs goals provide some detail concerning the content of the program and what is expected from the childcare worker; however, child goals provide a clear understanding of the outcomes expected for each individual child as a result of participating in the program.

## Child Goals

According to Peterson and Gunn (1984), a child goal is "a specific behavioral statement indicating a unit of knowledge or skill that the client is expected to accomplish" (p. 98). The purpose of establishing goals for individual children is to indicate the specific behavior that is to be achieved through participating in the program. This allows for the childcare worker to determine if progress is being made. One thing to note is that the child goals are more specific than program goals, in that the knowledge or skill is actually listed, giving the child a clear indication of the expected knowledge or skill to be achieved. Note the following child goal examples regarding the Social Interaction Skills program previously discussed:

> *Program Goal #1:* To teach the child to engage in conversation with peers, adults, and authority figures.
> *Child Goals:*
> 1. To introduce one's self to strangers appropriately.
> 2. To initiate a conversation with a peer.
> 3. To maintain eye contact with individuals who are speaking.
> 4. To listen when someone else is speaking.
>
> *Program Goal #2:* To teach the child methods of communicating effectively specific needs, wants, and requests for assistance.
> *Child Goals:*
> 1. To raise a hand when requesting assistance.
> 2. To use appropriate voice levels when indoors.
> 3. To use anger management skills when expressing anger.
> 4. To communicate assertively when expressing a need.

*Program Goal #3:* To instruct the child in engaging appropriately in dual and small group interactions.

*Child Goals:*

1. To share materials with peers in a small group interaction.
2. To compromise in order to reach an agreement with others.
3. To follow rules set by the group.
4. To display honesty in small group and dual interactions.
5. To contribute in cooperative group decision making.

*Program Goal #4:* To educate the child in the development of appropriate manners when with peers and authority figures in classroom, home, and community settings.

*Child Goals:*

1. To use the terms *please* and *thank you* when requesting a favor or assistance.
2. To display appropriate manners in various community settings.

*Program Goal #5:* To train the child to identify and utilize appropriate expression of emotions.

*Child Goals:*

1. To recognize age-appropriate expression of emotions when in the community and school setting.
2. To use an appropriate tone of voice when expressing anger and other negative feelings.
3. To monitor emotions on an ongoing basis.

The number of child goals depends on the complexity of the program and the needs of the children and youth. After child goals have been developed for the Social Interaction Skills program, it is necessary to develop more specific, outcome-oriented child objectives.

## Child Objectives

Child objectives are statements that outline the "exact behavior that will be taken as evidence" that the goals have been met by the child (Peterson and Gunn, 1984, p. 101). To state it another way, the purpose of the objective is to create a quantifiable measurement that will help the leader identify the child's progression or regression of a certain skill, ability, or knowledge area. The three parts to a child objective are labeled as follows:

- condition,
- behavior, and
- criteria.

The *condition* is *who, when, and where* the desired behavior will occur. This section is typically the first part mentioned when developing the child objective. The *behavior* portion of the child objective is very specific and *tells exactly what the child will do* to complete the objective. Peterson and Gunn (1984) note that the phrase "the child will" always should be included in the behavior section of a child objective, "followed by an action verb" (p. 105). Finally, the *criteria* section of the child objective specifies *to what extent* the behavior needs to take place. The criteria spells out to what extent the child must demonstrate completion before the objective has been met.

The following are some examples of the condition, behavior, and criteria that can be used when developing child objectives:

- *Condition:*
  - on request,
  - when with a peer,
  - during the social interaction skills program,
  - when faced with a problem,
  - upon discharge,
  - upon completion of the program, and
  - when asked;
- *Behavior:*
  - the child will name,
  - the child will state,
  - the child will write,
  - the child will choose,
  - the child will select, and
  - the child will introduce himself or herself;
- *Criteria:*
  - five out of seven times,
  - within one minute,
  - 100% of the time,
  - using proper form, and
  - one-fourth of the time.

The following are examples of child objectives that coordinate with the child goals previously mentioned. Note that the **condition** portion of the objective is in **bold** print, the *behavior* portion is in *italic* print, and the criteria portion is underlined for easier recognition of the components of the objective:

*Child Goal:* To share materials with peers in a small group interaction.
*Child Objectives:*
1. **Throughout the one-hour arts and crafts activity, and when requested by his peers,** the child *will pass* the scissors 90% of the time within 10 seconds of being asked, as recorded by the childcare worker.
2. **Throughout the one-hour arts and crafts activity,** the child *will return* all materials to be used by the group in the center of the table 100% of the time, as recorded by the childcare worker.

*Child Goal:* To compromise in order to reach an agreement with others.
*Child Objectives:*
1. **When faced with a conflict situation with a peer in the Cooperative Cooking class,** the child *will state* one positive conflict resolution technique that promotes cooperation, as approved by the childcare worker.
2. **During the Cooperative Cooking class, and when faced with a problem,** the child *will state* one solution that promotes compromise four out of five times, as judged by the childcare worker.

As with the child goals, it may be necessary to develop several child objectives to fully outline the expected conditions, behaviors, and criteria to be exhibited by the child. The objective should highlight the important parts of the behavior expected to show that he or she has succeeded at the task.

# Principle #2

*Only the children who need the program, should be placed in the program.*

For the specific program, Social Interaction Skills, to serve its purpose (assisting in the improvement, maintenance, and utilization of appropriate social interaction skills) the children, and *only* those children, who exhibit deficits regarding social interaction need to be placed in the program. Likewise, children who do not have social skill deficits should not be placed into the program. Implementing an assessment is a major essential component of intervention programming for at-risk youth. Dunn (1984) defined an assessment as "a systematic procedure for gathering select information about an individual for the purpose of making decisions regarding the individual's program or treatment plan" (p. 268). The assessment process will identify which children are appropriate to be involved in specific programs based on identified needs of each child. The assessment should focus on determining the level of skills, knowledge, and abilities of each client based on the goals established for the entire program.

Let us again consider the Social Interaction Skills program mentioned several times thus far. It has been determined that the Social Interaction Skills program will target five major goals during implementation. These are:

1. To encourage the child to engage in conversation with peers, adults, and authority figures.
2. To assist the child in communicating effectively specific needs, wants, and requests for assistance.
3. To aid the child in engaging appropriately in dual and small group interactions.
4. To assist the child in the development of appropriate manners when with peers and authority figures in classroom, home, and community settings.
5. To assist the child with the identification and appropriate expression of emotions.

Considering that these program goals are the focus of the specific program, it would make sense that the assessment identifies the child's deficits in these same areas. Therefore, the assessment should contain questions in the following areas regarding social interaction skills:

- child's ability to initiate conversation with peers, adults, and authority figures;
- child's ability to interact in dual and small group situations cooperatively;
- child's ability to request assistance, needs, and wants effectively;
- child's ability to display manners in home, classroom, and community settings; and
- child's ability to identify and express emotions appropriately.

When writing questions that are going to be included in the assessment, the childcare worker should refer back to the objectives that have been previously constructed to identify the exact expected behavior of the child. Let's consider the following objective:

*Objective:* When faced with a conflict situation with a peer in the Cooperative Cooking class, the child will state one positive conflict resolution technique that promotes cooperation, as approved by the childcare worker.

Since the objective states that the child needs to know conflict resolution skills to successfully participate in the activity, it only makes sense to observe the child *prior* to the program to determine if he or she has conflict resolution skills. This helps the childcare worker determine in which areas the child will need treatment and those in which he or she does not. Therefore, the childcare worker must refer to all objectives when writing assessment questions.

The following are possible assessment questions based on the previously mentioned objectives:

*Objective/Outcome:* When faced with a conflict situation with a peer in the Cooperative Cooking class, the child will state one positive conflict resolution technique that promotes cooperation, as approved by the childcare worker.
*Assessment Question:* Name one conflict resolution technique that promotes cooperation.

*Outcome/Objective:* During the Cooperative Cooking class, and when faced with a problem, the child will state one solution that promotes compromise four out of five times, as judged by the childcare worker.
*Assessment Question:* Name one way in which compromise can solve a problem.

*Outcome/Objective:* Throughout the one-hour arts and crafts activity, and when requested by his peers, the child will pass the scissors 90% of the time within 10 seconds of being asked, as recorded by the childcare worker.
*Assessment Question:* When a peer asks you to share an object, how do you react?

*Outcome/Objective:* Throughout the one-hour arts and crafts activity, the child will return all materials to be used by the group in the center of the table 100% of the time, as recorded by the childcare worker.
*Assessment Question:* When you are in an activity where sharing is important, state how you would handle the materials being used.

# Principle #3

*Only those activities that help create the best change should be used in the specific program.*

Once the specific program is developed, and the appropriate children are placed in the correct programs, selecting and analyzing which activities to use needs to take place. This process should be done for each program the childcare worker decides to create. The activities that are selected should provide assistance to the child with his or her achievement of the predetermined objectives. In order to determine if an activity will assist the child in meeting the predetermined objectives, a process called *activity analysis* is crucial.

## Activity Analysis

Activity analysis is "a procedure for breaking down and examining an activity's characteristics" (Peterson and Gunn, 1984, p. 180). In other words, activity analysis helps make sure the skills required for successful participation in the activity match the ability of the child. Specifically, activity analysis explores the physical, cognitive, social, and emotional requirements of the activity and determines the prerequisite skills, knowledge, and abilities demanded of the child. For example, if the child in the Social Interaction Skills program lacks the skills of reading and writing, then any activity involving the two behaviors should be modified or, if necessary, eliminated as possibilities for implementation. Again, the process of activity analysis aids in this determination and, as a result ensures intervention programming.

When determining the requirements of an activity, many elements need to be considered:

- *Physical:*
  - body position,
  - body parts,
  - types of movements,
  - coordination,
  - endurance,
  - hand-eye coordination, and
  - strength;
- *Cognitive:*
  - complexity of rules,
  - concentration,
  - memory, and
  - academic skills;
- *Social:*
  - social interaction patterns,
  - extent of physical contact,
  - levels of communication, and
  - number of children.
- *Emotional:*
  - joy,
  - guilt,
  - pain,
  - anger,
  - fear, and
  - frustration.

Activity analysis will tell a childcare worker which activities should be used in the program and which should not. An activity analysis compares the requirements of the activity (physical, social, intellectual, and emotional) with the skills of the children who are targeted to participate. If the children have the skills necessary to participate, then the activity may be appropriate for their involvement. If the children do not have the skills required by the activity, then the activity might be modified to meet the needs of the children. This process is known as activity modification.

## Activity Modification

Activity modification is a component of the activity analysis stage of specific program design. Since the activity analysis clearly defines the physical, cognitive, social, and emotional aspects of an activity, we then are able to "modify activities realistically and appropriately when needed" (Peterson and Gunn, 1984, p. 205). Peterson and Gunn (1984, p. 205) outlined some guidelines to consider when modifying activities:

1. Keep the activity and action close to the original or traditional activity.
2. Modify only those rules that need adapting.
3. Individualize the modification according to identified needs.
4. Do not always assume that an activity needs adapting.
5. When the child succeeds at the adapted activity, consider reevaluating the activity.
6. If the child is not succeeding at the adapted activity, consider another activity analysis.

For example, a childcare worker may decide to implement an activity that requires the use of various cognitive skills during the Social Interaction Skills program. The activity analysis process should have identified that the child needs reading and writing skills. In all other aspects, this activity is very appropriate. Since the assessment process found that a few of the children are unable to read or write, the leader will need to adapt the activity for those children. One way to do this may be by allowing the children to draw pictures rather than form sentences in order to get a thought across. This modification makes the necessary adaptations while allowing the activity to be successfully implemented.

Once the goals and objectives have been determined, the participants have been selected, and the activities have been analyzed, chosen and modified, the childcare worker is ready to lead the activity. However, planning does not stop there. A childcare worker must look at each activity in detail before, during and after implementation to determine effectiveness.

# Principle #4

*The activities chosen should be looked at in detail before, during, and after implementation to estimate how well they are assisting the child in creating a change.*

Once the activities have been selected, it is important that activity evaluation procedures are immediately put into action. According to Connolly (1984), evaluation measures are used to "identify program efficiency" and proving that the activity implemented did, indeed, create a change in the child's behavior. Connolly suggested that during evaluation, the childcare worker should ask the following questions:

- How well was the activity planned?
- How did the activity that was selected help the client meet his or her goals?
- Did the activity successfully aid the clients in meeting the client objectives?
- Did the content of the activity match the program goals?
- Was there enough staff?
- Was the activity too long?
- Was activity analysis performed?
- Was the activity modified appropriately and effectively?

In other words, the leader must evaluate all aspects of the program mentioned in this chapter to determine its effectiveness. Each individual child's progress also should be monitored following each activity to ensure the child objectives are being met. And, if not, the leader may be required to reanalyze the activities that are chosen through the activity analysis process. Or, a reevaluation of the child's goals and objectives may need to be considered.

# Summary

Overall, intervention-based programming is a complex process. However, with comprehensive decision making and efficient planning, a childcare worker can make a general recreation activity intervention in nature. If the childcare worker keeps in mind the four basic principles involved in intervention programming, a significant behavior change is more likely to occur in each individual child. As previously stated, a statement of purpose and program goals need to be developed. Once the overall structure of the program is determined, the development of child goals and objectives is essential in the planning process to determine the specific behavior changes that are expected of each child. It is also fundamentally important to remember that not *all* children are appropriate to participate in all programs. Therefore, an assessment must be developed and implemented to determine the specific needs of each child and which children should take part in each program.

When choosing specific activities that are going to be delivered to the children, the activity analysis step should never be overlooked in the planning process. It is crucial to determine the skills, knowledge, and abilities needed from each child participating in the activity and modifications should be developed on an individual basis accordingly.

Finally, the childcare worker is responsible for evaluating the effectiveness of the program and each activity before, during, and after activity implementation. If a childcare worker follows these principles and plans accordingly, a successful behavior change will likely occur.

# References

Connolly, P. (1984). Evaluation. In C. A. Peterson and S. L. Gunn, *Therapeutic recreation program design: Principles and procedures* (2nd ed.). Englewood Cliffs, NJ: Prentice-Hall, Inc.

Dunn, J. K. (1984). Assessment. In C. A. Peterson and S. L. Gunn, *Therapeutic recreation program design: Principles and procedures* (2nd ed.). Englewood Cliffs, NJ: Prentice-Hall, Inc.

Peterson, C. A., & Gunn, S. L. (1984). *Therapeutic recreation program design: Principles and procedures* (2nd ed.). Englewood Cliffs, NJ: Prentice-Hall, Inc.

# Chapter Three

# Intervention-Based Activity Resources

## by Sandra Larson

As mentioned in Chapter Two, it is important to select appropriate activities that will bring about the desired change of a child's behavior. Therefore, the purpose of this chapter is to provide a list of activity manuals and books that contain intervention-based activities that target specific goal areas. The following list of references has been categorized in the following manner:

- anger control and stress management;
- positive physical and mental health;
- cooperation, communication, and listening skills;
- problem-solving, decision-making, and planning skills;
- leisure awareness and leisure resources; and
- friendship and social skills.

An additional section has been added to outline specific Internet addresses that contain activities that can be adapted to target specific goals and target behaviors of a child.

## Anger Control and Stress Management

Bailey, R. V. (1992). *50 activities for managing stress.* Amherst, MA: HRD Press.

Bullaro, J. J. (1994). *Anger management: A manual of therapeutic activities.* San Pedro, CA: Difusco & Associates Wellness Program.

Cohen, M. J. (1993). *Well mind, well earth: 97 environmentally sensitive activities for stress management, spirit, and self-esteem.* Portland, OR: World Peace University.

Jones, A. (1996). *The wrecking ball of games and activities.* Ravensville, WA: Idyll Arbor, Inc.

Jones, A. (1998). *The wrecking ball of games and activities: Self-esteem, coping skills, communication, anger management, self-discovery, and teamwork.* Richland, WA: Rec. Room Publishing.

Schmidt, T. M. (1993). *Anger management and violence prevention: A group activities manual for middle- and high-school students.* Minneapolis, MN: Johnson Institute.

Toner, P. R. (1993). *Stress management and self-esteem activities.* West Nyack, NY: Center for Applied Research in Education.

Trower, T. (1995). *The self-control patrol workbook: Exercises for anger management.* King of Prussia, PA: Center for Applied Psychology.

## Positive Physical and Mental Health

Bittinger, G. (1994). *Teaching snacks: Teaching basic concepts and skills through cooking.* Everett, WA: Warren Publishing House.

Catalano, C. (1994). *The fit kids collection: Aerobic fitness and skill activities for preschool through sixth grade children.* Seattle, WA: Fit Kids.

Delisle, D. (1996). *Growing good kids: 28 activities to enhance self-awareness, compassion, and leadership.* Minneapolis, MN: Free Spirit Publishers.

Harrison, J. C. (1996). *Hooked on fitness! Fun physical conditioning games and activities for grades K–8.* New York, NY: Prentice-Hall, Inc.

Huff, P. (1992). *The cooperative indoor and outdoor game book: Easy classroom and field games for fitness and fun.* New York, NY: Scholastic, Inc.

Jones, A. (1996). *The wrecking ball of games and activities.* Ravensville, WA: Idyll Arbor, Inc.

Jones, A. (1998). *The wrecking ball of games and activities: Self-esteem, coping skills, communication, anger management, self-discovery, and teamwork.* Richland, WA: Rec. Room Publishing.

# Cooperation, Communication, and Listening

Bittinger, G. (1994). *Teaching snacks: Teaching basic concepts and skills through cooking.* Everett, WA: Warren Publishing House.

Bittinger, G. (1996). *Bear hugs for getting along: Positive activities that encourage cooperation and sharing.* Everett, WA: Warren Publishing House.

Brown, M. (1990). *Activities for cooperative learning: Group projects, art, social skills, problem solving, writing, and games.* Huntington Beach, CA: Teacher Created Materials.

Goodman, J. M. (1992). *Group solutions: Cooperative logic activities.* Berkeley, CA: Great Explorations in Math and Science.

Goodman, J. M. (1997). *Group solutions, too! More cooperative logic activities for grades K–4.* Berkeley, CA: Great Explorations in Math and Science.

Huff, P. (1992). *The cooperative indoor and outdoor game book: Easy classroom and field games for fitness and fun.* New York, NY: Scholastic, Inc.

Jones, A. (1996). *The wrecking ball of games and activities.* Ravensville, WA: Idyll Arbor, Inc.

Jones, A. (1998). *The wrecking ball of games and activities: Self-esteem, coping skills, communication, anger management, self-discovery, and teamwork.* Richland, WA: Rec. Room Publishing.

Palim, J. (1996). *Jamboree: Communication activities for children.* Harlow, UK: Longman.

Schilling, D. (1993). *Getting along: Activities for teaching cooperation, responsibility, and respect.* Spring Valley, CA: Innerchoice Publishing.

Wenc, C. C. (1993). *Cooperation: Learning through laughter: 51 brief activities for groups of all ages.* Minneapolis, MN: Educational Media Corp.

# Problem-Solving, Decision-Making, and Planning Skills

Brown, M. (1990). *Activities for cooperative learning: Group projects, art, social skills, problem solving, writing, and games.* Huntington Beach, CA: Teacher Created Materials.

Elwell, P. A. (1993). *CPS for teens: Classroom activities for teaching creative problem solving.* Waco, TX: Prufrock.

Jones, A. (1996). *The wrecking ball of games and activities.* Ravensville, WA: Idyll Arbor, Inc.

Jones, A. (1998). *The wrecking ball of games and activities: Self-esteem, coping skills, communication, anger management, self-discovery, and teamwork.* Richland, WA: Rec. Room Publishing.

Landin, L. (1996). *Mind treks: Creative, hands-on problem-solving activities.* Parsippany, NJ: Fearon Teacher Aids.

Landin, L. (1996). *More mind treks: Creative, hands-on problem solving: Grades 4–6.* Parsippany, NJ: Fearon Teacher Aids.

Landin, L. (1997). *Mind treks III: Creative, hands-on problem-solving activities.* Parsippany, NJ: Fearon Teacher Aids.

Perry, C. (1994). *Thinking it through: Activities to develop good thinking skills.* Melbourne, Australia: Oxford University Press.

# Leisure Awareness

Stumbo, N. J., & Thompson, S. R. (1990). *Leisure education: Activities and resources.* State College, PA: Venture Publishing, Inc.

Stumbo, N. J. (1992). *Leisure Education II: More activities and resources.* State College, PA: Venture Publishing, Inc.

Stumbo, N. J. (1997). *Leisure Education III: More goal-oriented activities.* State College, PA: Venture Publishing, Inc.

Stumbo, N. J. (1998). *Leisure Education IV: Activities for individuals with substance addictions.* State College, PA: Venture Publishing, Inc.

# Social Skills and Friendship Building

Brown, M. (1990). *Activities for cooperative learning: Group projects, art, social skills, problem solving, writing, and games.* Huntington Beach, CA: Teacher Created Materials.

Dixon, D. A. (1990). *Teaching young children to care: 37 activities for developing concern for others.* Mystic, CT: Twenty-Third Publications.

Fox, L. C. (1993). *Let's get together: Activities for developing friendship and self-esteem in the elementary grades: Affiliation/belongingness techniques that work.* Rolling Hills Estates, CA: Jalmar Press.

Heyne, L. A. (1994). *Making friends: Using recreation activities to promote friendship between children with and without disabilities.* Minneapolis, MN: School of Kinesiology and Leisure Studies.

Jones, A. (1996). *The wrecking ball of games and activities.* Ravensville, WA: Idyll Arbor, Inc.

Jones, A. (1998). *The wrecking ball of games and activities: Self-esteem, coping skills, communication, anger management, self-discovery, and teamwork.* Richland, WA: Rec. Room Publishing.

Mannix, D. (1993). *Social skills activities for special children.* West Nyack, NY: Center for Applied Research in Education.

Mannix, D. (1998). *Social skills activities for secondary learners with special needs.* West Nyack, NY: Center for Applied Research in Education.

Schmidt, J. J. (1997). *Making and keeping friends: Ready-to-use lessons, stories, and activities for building relationships (grades 4–8).* West Nyack, NY: Center for Applied Research in Education.

Schilling, D. (1996). *50 activities for teaching emotional intelligence.* Spring Valley, CA: Innerchoice Publishing.

Wade, R. C. (1991). *Joining hands: From personal to planetary friendship in the primary classroom.* Tucson, AZ: Zephyr Press.

# Anger Control and Stress Management

# Rap Sheet

**Space Requirements:** Activity room

**Equipment/Resource Requirements:** Paper, writing utensils, tape player, background music, example of rap song

**Group Size:** Small or large group

**Program Goals:**
1. To increase participants' ability to generate alternative solutions to fighting.
2. To allow participants to express themselves in a medium that may be appropriate to their interests.

**Program Description:**
**Preparation:**
The leader should provide an example of a rap song for individuals who may be unfamiliar with that type of song.

**Introduction:**
The purpose of this activity is to help participants generate alternatives to fighting. The leader should explain that there is no logical reason to submit to physical fights at any time. The leader should explain that there is always a way out, always a better solution.

**Activity Description:**
The leader directs the participants to break up into small groups (three to five persons per group). Each group is given 15 minutes to write a rap song about what to do instead of fighting.

The participants should be encouraged to contribute equally to the song. Next, the small groups present their rap songs to the whole group. Finally, the leader should use the following questions to end the activity.

**Debriefing Questions/Closure:**
1. How did it feel to put such a basic concept as not fighting into a rap song?
2. How did you participate individually? How did you participate as a group?
3. How did it feel to rap in front of the group?
4. How well do you think your message got across?
5. What did you learn about alternatives to fighting?

**Leadership Considerations:**
1. The leader should make sure that lyrics are appropriate.
2. The leader should make sure all participants are contributing to the best of their ability.

**Variations:**
1. Music is a great way for children to learn. This activity can be adapted into a role-play of events.
2. The leader can provide instruments for the participants to play.

**Creator:** Kristen Boys, Illinois State University, Normal, Illinois.

# Emotions Puppets

**Space Requirements:** Classroom or activity room

**Equipment/Resource Requirements:** Two paper plates per participant, different colors of construction paper, glue, scissors, one Popsicle stick per participant, stapler, markers, various craft supplies appropriate for decorating a face

**Group Size:** Small group

**Program Goals:**
1. To increase participants' ability to illustrate and discuss emotions.
2. To increase participants' ability to distinguish between different emotions.

**Program Description:**
**Preparation:**
The leader should have a completed example to show to the group.

**Introduction:**
The purpose of this activity is to help participants distinguish between emotions. The leader should explain to the group members that they will be constructing paper plate puppets.

**Activity Description:**
The leader instructs participants to sit at the table. The leader explains to the participants that they can use any of the supplies on the table to decorate their puppets. Each side of the puppet should reflect a different emotion.

Once each participant has both plates decorated, the leader instructs the participants to staple the two paper plates together, having a face showing on each side. They then glue a Popsicle stick between the plates at the bottom of the puppets. The puppets can now be used as a way for each individual to show how he or she may feel.

After everyone has completed this step, the leader initiates a discussion on emotions. The discussion should touch upon various emotions that people typically feel and the conditions under which they are normally felt. Each person in the group should tell a story that involves the emotions displayed on his or her puppet. During his or her storytelling he or she can use the puppets to express the emotion that was felt.

The activity ends with the leader reemphasizing the goals, using the following debriefing questions.

**Debriefing Questions/Closure:**
1. How do you describe an emotion?
2. How are emotions helpful?
3. What are some reasons it's important to identify your emotions?
4. How does a person who is happy look?
5. How does a person who is sad look?
6. What are positive emotions versus not so positive emotions?
7. How do you normally show your emotions?
8. Why are emotions important?

**Leadership Considerations:**
1. The leader should make sure everyone is comfortable in sharing a story with the group.
2. The leader may set an example by sharing a story first.

**Variations:**
1. The leader may allow each individual to choose what emotions his or her puppet will represent and then have the group guess what each one is.
2. The leader may have the puppet faces reflect the emotions the participants feel when they are participating in a leisure activity of their choice or when they face leisure barriers.

**Creator:** Jennifer Matkowich, Illinois State University, Normal, Illinois.

# Stress Balls

**Space Requirements:** Classroom or activity room

**Equipment/Resource Requirements:** Balloons, paper funnels, and Styrofoam cups (one of each for each participant); one to two pounds of sand, several newspapers or large tarp to cover work area

**Group Size:** Small group

**Program Goals:**
1. To increase participants' awareness of the sources of stress.
2. To teach participants one way to reduce stress.
3. To help participants create a tool that can aid in reducing stress.

**Program Description:**
**Preparation:**
Prior to beginning the activity, the leader should place newspapers on top of the working area, to avoid a mess when making the stress balls. All of the needed supplies should be arranged in the middle of the work area.

**Introduction:**
The purpose of this activity is to increase participants' awareness of stress, to teach participants one way to reduce stress, and to create a tool that can aid in reducing or relieving stress.

The leader begins the activity by asking the group members if they know what stress is. Each participant is given an opportunity to explain his or her definition of stress.

A suggestion for beginning the activity is as follows:

Today we are going to talk about stress. Can anyone give me an example of what stress is? What are some of the things that happen to our body when a stressful situation arises? How do you deal with stress? We are going to make what is called *a stress ball*. This ball can be used to massage the fingers and can be gripped when an individual feels stress. Please wait your turn as materials are passed out.

**Activity Description:**
The leader will ask the participants to sit around the table. Each participant will be given a balloon and a paper funnel. The leader will distribute one cup of sand to each participant. The participants will be instructed to fill their balloons with the sand by using the paper funnel.

To fill the balloon, each participant needs to take the end of the balloon and fit it over the mouth of the funnel. The sand then is poured into the funnel to fill the balloon (use only about one cup of sand per balloon). The participant should tie off his or her balloon. The participants now have created their own stress ball.

The leader should use the following debriefing questions to close the activity. The leader should also reiterate the purpose of the activity.

The leader may ask the participants to help clean up the area and put away supplies after the debriefing questions.

**Debriefing Questions/Closure:**
1. Test your stress ball once by squeezing it. How does it feel?
2. How do you think this will help you to deal with stress and anger?
3. Describe times when you have felt stressed.
4. How did stress feel? What were clues you were under stress?
5. What are some other physical or mental ways you think you could manage stress?
6. Which of these have you used before?
7. Which of these can you use in the future?

**Leadership Considerations:**
1. The leader should allow the participants to create a stress ball on their own and assist only if requested. This is typically a messy activity; however, it is highly encouraged that each individual be in control of making his or her own stress ball.
2. If participants appear to have difficulty in identifying what stress is and its related symptoms, the leader should be prepared with several examples that are at participants' knowledge and experience level.

**Variations:**
1. Instead of using sand to fill the balloon, the leader may choose to use salt or rice as an alternative.
2. The leader may choose to do this as a follow-up activity after a session on stress and/or stress management.

**Creator:** Amy Conron, Illinois State University, Normal, Illinois.

# Recipe for Success

**Space Requirements:** Classroom or activity room

**Equipment/Resource Requirements:** Blank note cards, pencils, pens, small plastic or cardboard boxes

**Group Size:** Small group

**Program Goals:**
1. To increase participants' awareness of the concept of anger management.
2. To increase participants' awareness of the importance of anger management.
3. To increase participants' knowledge of anger management techniques.

**Program Description:**
**Preparation:**
The leader may have participants bring in their own boxes or try to have them donated.

**Introduction:**
The leader explains that the purpose of this activity is to increase awareness of positive versus aggressive situations.

**Activity Description:**
The leader begins by explaining to the group what anger management is and why it is important to use anger management techniques. Next, the leader gives the group some examples of anger management techniques (e.g., relaxation, exercises, and counting to 10). After giving an example, the leader asks participants to define the term *aggression* in their own words. Last, the leader asks participants to recall a situation where they had difficulty in controlling their anger. They should discuss the antecedents, behavior, and consequences.

Following the discussion, the leader gives each participant several blank note cards. The leader explains that they should come up with scenarios in which a stressful situation may take place (i.e., taking other's personal property without asking). For each scenario, participants are encouraged to come up with three different ways to avoid or deal with that aggressive situation.

After everyone has completed his or her note cards, the problems and solutions note cards are placed in the small box. This then can be used as a reference for future use. (Box and setup should resemble a file folder or recipe box.) The leader explains to participants that they now have a reference to look at when needing a solution to an aggressive situation.

The leader ends the activity by discussing the following debriefing questions. The discussion should focus on the purpose of the activity.

**Debriefing Questions/Closure:**
1. When are we most likely to get angry?
2. Describe a situation where you didn't handle your anger well. Look for antecedents, behavior, and consequences.
3. Describe a situation where you did manage your anger well. Again, look for antecedents, behavior, and consequences.
4. What are some alternatives for managing your anger?
5. What technique will you try this week?

**Leadership Considerations:**
1. The leader should have some examples of aggressive problems and solutions made ahead of time.
2. The leader should be prepared to give a detailed and easy-to-understand definition of aggression.
3. The leader should have all participants read their cards to the group.

**Variations:**
1. The leader may change the content from aggression to leisure resources, leisure barriers, or stress management.

2. Instead of doing this on note cards, the leader may write problems and solutions on a large banner that can be placed on a wall where everyone can see it at all times.

**Creator:** Sandra Larson, Illinois State University, Normal, Illinois.

# What Do You Do When You're Stressed Out or Angry?

**Spacing Requirements:** Classroom or activity room

**Equipment/Resource Requirements:** Blankets or mats to lie on

**Group Size:** Small group

**Program Goals:**
1. To increase participants' knowledge of anger control.
2. To increase participants' knowledge of relaxation techniques.

**Program Description:**

**Preparation:**
The leader will place mats on the floor in a circle ahead of time. The activity should take place in a quiet place with no distractions.

**Introduction:**
The purpose of this activity is to assist participants in identifying how they most typically deal with anger. It will also show participants alternative ways to relax.

A suggestion for introducing the activity is as follows:

> We are going to talk about ways to control our anger. Can someone give an example of when he or she was angry? What do you do if you become angry? We are going to go around the circle, so everyone think of a situation where you have been angry.

**Activity Description:**
The participants sit in a circle on the mats. This makes a great formation for discussion. The leader asks the participants if they would like to share a situation when they have been angry. The leader then asks them what they do when they are angry. Do they have a tantrum, stomp away,

or punch walls? After each person has given an answer, the leader demonstrates the different anger releasing techniques:

> *First Technique*—Tense every muscle in your body for 10 seconds and then release. Do this a couple times.

> *Second Technique*—Sit up, close your eyes and count to 10. After that try and count from 10 backwards with your eyes closed. Make sure you are not counting too fast.

> *Third Technique*—Lay back on the mat and close your eyes. Picture your favorite place or favorite food (each participant can describe these items if he or she wants). When you get angry you can think about these favorite things.

Once all techniques have been practiced, the techniques are discussed by the group. The discussion should focus on the importance of releasing anger in appropriate ways.

**Debriefing Questions/Closure:**
1. Name an event in everyday life that makes you upset.
2. What is an example of a little thing that can make you upset?
3. Why is it good to control your anger?
4. What would happen if everyone lashed out when he or she was angry?
5. What are three ways we learned today to help us manage our anger?

**Leadership Considerations:**
1. The leader should make sure the participants are not accusing each other in their examples.
2. The leader should make sure the mats have plenty of space between them.

3. Some participants may not be comfortable with sharing angry situations, as the situations may be private moments.

**Variations:**
1. The participants can role-play situations.
2. The participants can make up their own relaxation techniques and teach them to the rest of the group.

**Creator:** Courtney Stauffer, Illinois State University, Normal, Illinois.

# Conflict Resolution

**Space Requirements:** Classroom or activity room

**Equipment/Resource Requirements:** Poster with four-step conflict resolution process listed and tape or blackboard and chalk, various scenarios of conflict

**Group Size:** Small group

**Program Goals:**
1. To improve participants' effective dual conversation skills.
2. To improve participants' ability to resolve conflicts.
3. To allow participants the opportunity to exercise conflict resolution skills.

**Program Description:**
**Preparation:**
The leader gathers and prepares materials. The poster is taped to the wall.

**Introduction:**
The leader explains to the participants that they will practice new ways to resolve conflicts with other individuals through a four-step process. Participants will be asked to chose a partner and role-play after a brief discussion.

**Activity Description:**
The leader explains to the group a variety of methods that can be used as conflict resolution (i.e., talk the problem out, walk away from the individual, ignore the problem and move on, find someone who can help). Next, the leader will explain to the group that for this particular activity a four-step conflict resolution process will be followed. The four steps include:

1. recognize a conflict is present;
2. write down, or mentally note, emotions and reactions;
3. analyze the emotions and reactions; and
4. choose an appropriate method of resolution according to the setting and circumstances.

At this point, the participants will take turns role-playing to practice conflict resolution (e.g., a bully at school). Each participant will get one turn to practice the four-step approach to resolve the conflict while another participant acts as the aggressor. During this time the leader will watch the participants and offer suggestions of additional ways to handle the situation. The process is repeated using various scenarios until everyone has had an opportunity to play both roles.

The leader ends the activity by discussing the following questions. *Note:* Other questions and discussions may arise which should be addressed. The leader should remind participants of the four steps involved in the process they learned for conflict resolution.

**Debriefing Questions/Closure:**
1. When does conflict occur?
2. What are appropriate ways to resolve conflicts?
3. What are inappropriate ways to resolve conflicts?
4. What is the four-step process we learned here today?
5. How did you feel in the various role-plays?
6. What did you learn concerning conflict resolution?
7. How will what was learned today assist you in the future?

**Leadership Considerations:**
1. The leader should use age-appropriate situations such as school, work, or athletics.
2. The leader needs to be adequately prepared with a variety of situations.

3. The leader needs to be aware and cautious of individuals who may be prone to using physical violence.

**Variations:**

1. The leader may have scenarios written on cards that present conflicts and have groups of two come up with potential resolutions.

2. The leader may focus more on the actual resolution than the method of resolving a conflict.

**Creator:** Craig W. Strohbeck, Illinois State University, Normal, Illinois.

# Leisure as an Aggression Reducer

**Space Requirements:** Classroom or activity room

**Equipment/Resource Requirements:** Homemade Wheel of Fortune Game, dry erase board, markers, and prizes (if desired)

**Group Size:** Small group

**Program Goals:**
1. To increase participants' awareness of typical personality traits of an aggressor.
2. To promote leisure as a way of redirecting aggressive feelings.
3. To teach participants positive solutions to aggressive situations.

**Program Description:**
**Preparation:**
Categories:

1. Personality traits of aggressive people
2. Leisure activities
3. Positive solutions to aggressive situations

The leader writes all the letters of the alphabet on the dry erase board and has the phrases written on note cards; for example:

*Personality Traits:*
- short-tempered,
- bullies,
- angry, and
- unhappy.

*Leisure Activities:*
- computer games,
- chess,
- watching television, and
- playing soccer.

*Positive Solutions:*
- compromise,
- walk away,
- negotiate,
- cooperate, and
- exercise.

**Introduction:**
The leader explains to the participants that they will be playing a modified form of Wheel of Fortune. The three categories are listed and the leader explains that the participants will need to choose letters from the alphabet. If the letter chosen is a letter in the puzzle phrase, the letter will be exposed and that individual will get another turn.

**Activity Description:**
The leader explains that the game will be played as it is on television, following the same rules of the television game show. Each participant will play individually.

After each puzzle is solved, the leader holds a discussion outlining the importance of each. The game should be played until all puzzles have been solved or until time runs out. The focus is on the potential of leisure as an aggression reducer.

**Debriefing Questions/Closure:**
1. What are characteristics of aggressive people?
2. How do aggressive people behave or act?
3. What are consequences of being aggressive?
4. How can leisure activities help reduce feelings of aggression?
5. What other solutions are there to reducing aggression?
6. How will you reduce aggression next time?

**Leadership Considerations:**
1. The leader should make sure participants are able to read.
2. The leader should make sure participants understand rules of Wheel of Fortune.

**Variation:**
The leader should use appropriate content for puzzles.

**Creator:** Sandra Larson, Illinois State University, Normal, Illinois.

# Move to the Music

**Space Requirements:** Large room with open space

**Equipment/Resource Requirements:** Cassette or CD player and cassettes or CDs including music by Mozart; the soundtracks to *The Lion King, The Little Mermaid,* and *Aladdin;* and oldies music

**Group Size:** Small group

**Program Goals:**
1. To increase participants' knowledge of stress.
2. To increase participants' ability to verbalize stress within their daily life.
3. To increase participants' ability to use stress management skills in relation to creative movements.

**Program Description:**

**Preparation:**
The leader should have music taped on a cassette ahead of time. Also, the stretches should be planned.

**Introduction:**
The purpose of this activity is to provide participants with the opportunity to increase knowledge of stress, verbalize stress within their daily life, and provide the opportunity to utilize stress management techniques in relation to creative movement.

**Activity Description:**
The leader will state the goals and purpose of the activity. Participants will begin by sitting within the outlined circle in the center of the room. A short discussion will be held on what stress is, how one feels when one is stressed, and areas of stress within the participants' lives.

The leader will state directions for the activity. Participants will choose an area that is their own personal space (which was previously defined in the directions) throughout the room. This will allow each participant to move freely without disturbing others.

A slow song will be played first to allow the participants to stretch out tense muscles and warmup.

Participants will stretch each muscle in their body beginning with the neck and moving to the ankles. Stretches will be held for 15–30 seconds.

Music will be played and participants will be instructed to concentrate only on the music and move creatively to the beat. When the music stops, the participants will freeze until the next piece of music is played. A variety of music will be played including slow and upbeat to allow participants to get lost in the music.

A slow classical song will be played to allow the participants to slowly wind down. Participants should be instructed to repeat previous stretching sequence to stretch muscles. Participants should also be told to breathe deeply by inhaling and exhaling slowly.

A discussion will be held to discuss the different songs that might have caused stress or relieved stress and how the music made the participants feel. Also, other activities to relieve stress will be discussed.

The leader will restate the goals and purpose of the activity.

**Debriefing Questions/Closure:**
1. What is stress?
2. How do you feel when you experience stress?
3. What are some areas of stress in your life?
4. How did the music make you feel?
5. What types of music were the most relaxing and enjoyable?
6. Which types of music caused anxiety?
7. What types of music would you listen to if you wanted to relax?
8. Which other activities can you participate in to take you away from stress in your life?

**Leadership Considerations:**

1. It may be important to choose music carefully because of the effects it may have on the participants' mood or behavior.
2. The leader should state that almost any type of movement is acceptable for the activity, and demonstrate some movements. However, boundaries should be set that inform participants of inappropriate actions to prevent the possibility of a participant touching or hitting another participant, for example.
3. Participants may need prompting by providing indirect suggestions for types of movement for some types of music.

**Variations:**

1. Cognitive skills could be implemented to the activity by having participants learn rhythm skills. First, participants would be taught what rhythm is, and practice by marching, clapping, and moving the head, arms, and feet to the beat of the music. If participants are able to grasp the concept, different types of music could then be played and participants will have to move to the varying rhythms.
2. Physical endurance can be highlighted by leading the activity for five minutes without stopping, and increasing the time limit by two minutes each week.
3. Cooperative skills can be emphasized by having the participant paired with another participant doing mirror imaging. The activity would be run in a similar manner. However, when the music is played, the first participant would be the leader, and the second participant would have to follow. When the song changed, the second participant would be the leader.

**Creator:** Renee Raczkowski, Illinois State University, Normal, Illinois.

# Paint to the Music

**Space Requirements:** Classroom or activity room

**Equipment/Resource Requirements:** Stereo, cassette(s), paints, paintbrushes, watercolor paper, cups for rinse water, clean-up supplies

**Group Size:** Small group

**Program Goals:**
1. To improve participants' ability to relieve stress through painting to music.
2. To provide participants with opportunity to increase self-expression in art and music.

**Program Description:**
**Preparation:**
The leader will prepare a tape of appropriate music to play and gather supplies ahead of time.

**Introduction:**
The purpose of this activity is to increase participants' ability to manage stress through painting to music.

**Activity Description:**
The leader begins the activity by stating the goals and purpose of the activity. A discussion on the importance of relieving stress is held. The participants also will discuss what colors and shapes typically represent certain sounds or moods.

The leader will give instructions for the activity, telling the participants that they will create a painting that expresses how the music makes them feel. When the music begins, the participants will take their paintbrushes, dip it in the color of their choice and begin to paint.

Different songs will be played to reflect different moods. When the music stops, they are to put their paintbrushes down and wait for the next song to be played.

When the music begins again, they have the option of choosing another color after rinsing their brushes. Participants should be encouraged to be creative with their artwork and to paint with colors and shapes relating to how the music makes them feel. The participants should be reminded to keep the paint on the paper, and to rinse their brushes each time they change colors.

The leader should give the participants the opportunity to share and discuss their paintings. They may discuss the reasons why they chose different colors and shapes for the different types of music.

The purpose of the activity should be restated. Debriefing questions can be used for closure.

**Debriefing Questions/Closure:**
1. What is stress?
2. What are different ways to relieve stress?
3. What music did you like best as a stress reliever?
4. How did your painting reflect your feelings?
5. How does art help relieve stress?
6. How can you use this in the future?

**Leadership Considerations:**
1. The leader should remind participants to work on following directions.
2. The leader should encourage participants to be creative with their work and paint with colors and shapes relating to how the music makes them feel.
3. The leader should remind participants to keep the paint on the paper and to rinse their brushes each time they change colors.

**Variations:**
1. The leader may choose to play the music and have the participants move their paintbrushes to the rhythm of the music.
2. For individuals who cannot handle paint, markers or crayons can be used.

**Creator:** Renee Raczkowski, Illinois State University, Normal, Illinois.

# Putting the Pieces Back Together

**Space Requirements:** Classroom or activity room

**Equipment/Resource Requirements:** Squares of poster board or cardboard, markers, plastic bags for pieces, scissors

**Group Size:** Small group

**Program Goals:**
1. To increase participants' knowledge of anger.
2. To increase participants' ability to verbally express situations in which they get angry.
3. To increase participants' ability to identify appropriate alternatives to expressing anger.

**Program Description:**
**Preparation:**
The leader should cut the poster board or cardboard into approximately 5-by-7-inch squares.

**Introduction:**
The purpose of this activity is to provide participants with the opportunity to increase their knowledge of, and ability to verbally anger express, while identifying appropriate alternatives to expressing anger.

**Activity Description:**
The leader begins the activity by stating the goals and purpose of the activity. A discussion about what anger is and in what situations participants get angry is held. The leader gives instructions for the activity.

The leader instructs each participant to draw a picture of himself or herself participating in a leisure activity he or she enjoys. The participants are told that these pictures will be cut into puzzle pieces. The leader distributes materials.

One piece will be cut from the picture each time a participant states a situation in which he or she gets angry. When about half of the 5-by-7-inch square has been cut into pieces, the participant will then cut one piece from the picture each time he or she can describe an appropriate way of expressing anger.

The leader allows participants to think of ideas while drawing their leisure picture.

Each participant is paired with another child to trade puzzles and help each other put them together. The leader holds a discussion on the importance of expressing anger appropriately, and the importance of others' help.

The leader restates the goals of the activity. Discussion questions are useful to refocus on participants' goals.

**Debriefing Questions/Closure:**
1. How do you feel when you feel angry?
2. What are appropriate ways to express anger?
3. What are inappropriate ways to express anger?
4. How can leisure activities help you reduce or express anger?
5. What will you do the next time you're angry?

**Leadership Considerations:**
1. The leader encourages participants to listen to others and speak when it is their turn.
2. The leader provides suggestions to assist participants in their responses.
3. The leader encourages participants to be courteous in order to make others feel comfortable, and be able to freely express their emotions.

**Variations:**
1. This activity may be used as a stress management activity.
2. This activity may also be used for dealing with feelings, for instance, what others do that hurt their feelings.
3. To decrease levels of frustration, precut puzzles should be used with younger children or those who have difficulty using scissors.

**Creator:** Renee Raczkowski, Illinois State University, Normal, Illinois.

# Learning to Visualize and Relax

**Space Requirements:** Classroom or activity room

**Equipment/Resource Requirements:** Soft music, cassette player, comfortable room with pillows, personal space

**Group Size:** Small group

**Program Goals:**
1. To improve participants' awareness of personal relaxation techniques.
2. To improve participants' ability to identify personal areas of stress.
3. To improve participants' ability to utilize relaxation and visualization techniques.

**Program Description:**
**Preparation:**
The leader can purchase or prepare a relaxation tape. The leader should write a visualization script (or locate a prepared one). The environment should be as soothing as possible.

**Introduction:**
The purpose of this activity is to provide participants with an opportunity to control personal stress, manage it successfully within their lives, and create a personal plan for relaxation.

**Activity Description:**
The leader should state goals and the purpose of the activity. The leader explains how relaxation and visualization are beneficial for managing stress. The leader asks the participants to identify sources of stress within their lives. What do they currently do to help manage that stress?

The leader plays the music and allows the participants to get comfortable within their personal space. The leader then will describe colors, places, and feelings for the participants to imagine independently. After participants are fully relaxed, the leader will ask them to get up slowly and end their personal relaxation.

The leader should restate the goals and purpose of the activity and let the participants comment about what they learned. The following debriefing questions can assist with closure.

**Debriefing Questions/Closure:**
1. What are sources of stress for you?
2. What actions do you take to manage that stress?
3. How can relaxation tapes help reduce your stress?
4. How can visualization techniques help reduce your stress?
5. How might you incorporate either of these techniques into your daily life?
6. What did you learn today that you can use in the future?

**Leadership Considerations:**
1. The leader should make sure the environment is inviting, relaxing, and comforting.
2. The leader should make sure the visualization is one participants can relate to.

**Variations:**
1. The leader may change the music to create different moods.
2. The leader may change the visualization script to create different moods.

**Creator:** Monika Ressel, Illinois State University, Normal, Illinois.

# Feelings Sculptures

**Space Requirements:** Classroom or activity room

**Equipment/Resource Requirements:** Modeling clay or dough, prerecorded tape of different types of music

**Group Size:** Small group

**Program Goals:**
1. To improve participants' ability to identify and express personal feelings.
2. To improve participants' ability to recognize different types of music that make them feel specific ways, and may be used for stress management.

**Program Description:**

**Preparation:**
The leader will gather supplies and prepare tape of music.

**Introduction:**
The purpose of this activity is to help participants identify and express personal feelings and recognize that music may be used for stress management.

**Activity Description:**
The leader begins by stating the goals and purpose of the activity. The group will discuss different emotions experienced by the participants. The leader will distribute materials to all participants and instruct participants not to begin sculpting material until the music begins. Several different types and tempos of music will be played.

After each type of music, the participants will discuss their sculptures with the group. Discussion should include what the participants made and how the music made them feel.

The leader should encourage the participants to express themselves however they feel most comfortable.

The leader should restate the goals and purpose of the activity and let the group members comment about their individual and unique feelings. Use the following debriefing questions.

**Debriefing Questions/Closure:**
1. Does everyone have emotions or feelings?
2. What purpose do emotions serve? Why do we have them?
3. Which type of music did you like the best?
4. How does your sculpture reflect your feelings?
5. How can identifying your emotions help to manage stress?
6. What should you do when you're happy? What about when you are sad, bored, excited, upset, or scared?

**Leadership Considerations:**
1. Participants may want to use separate pieces of clay for each type of music.
2. The leader should establish a safe and comfortable environment.

**Variation:**
The participants may use other media besides clay.

**Creator:** Monika Ressel, Illinois State University, Normal, Illinois.

# The Stress-Free Ladder

**Space Requirements:** Classroom or activity room

**Equipment/Resource Requirements:** Accompanying work sheet, pencils, balloons, sand, funnel

**Group Size:** Small group

**Program Goals:**
1. To improve participants' awareness of life situations that are stressful.
2. To improve participants' ability to identify ways that will help them to reduce or manage their stress.
3. To provide participants with an opportunity to make an object that they will be able to use in future stressful situations.

**Program Description:**

**Preparation:**
The leader will make one copy of the work sheet per participant. The leader will fill one balloon with a cup of sand as an example of a stress ball.

**Introduction:**
The purpose of this activity is to provide participants with the opportunity to express personal ideas about stress within their lives and create a way that can help manage stress in the future.

**Activity Description:**
The leader should state the goals and the purpose of the activity. Participants are asked to identify situations that are stressful to them. The leader should explain the ladder exercise and distribute work sheets and pencils.

Starting at the bottom rung, the participants should identify ways to reduce stress in their lives. Possible ways and ideas include saying no, listening to music, talking to friends, exercising, practicing yoga, staying active, eating right, and simplifying. The leader should assist participants in writing down things that help them control stress in their personal lives. Starting at the bottom, the participants will work their way up the ladder with various ways to reduce or manage stress.

After the work sheets are completed, the leader introduces the stress ball activity and shows the example. The leader distributes materials and assists participants in making their own personal stress balls. The leader discusses how handling the stress ball could help get rid of stressful energy.

The leader should restate the goals and purpose of the activity and let the group members comment on what they learned.

**Debriefing Questions/Closure:**
1. Name three constructive ways to reduce or manage your stress.
2. What new ways to manage stress did you hear today?
3. Why is it important to reduce or manage stress?
4. What would life be like with no stress?
5. When can stress be good for you? When can stress be bad for you?
6. What new way to manage stress will you use tomorrow?

**Leadership Considerations:**
1. This activity requires considerable cognitive ability.
2. The leader may have stress balls already made if activity with sand would be too messy.

**Variation:**
The ladder may be used as a way to look at leisure preferences, leisure barriers, and social skills.

**Creator:** Monika Ressel, Illinois State University, Normal, Illinois.

# The Stress-Free Ladder

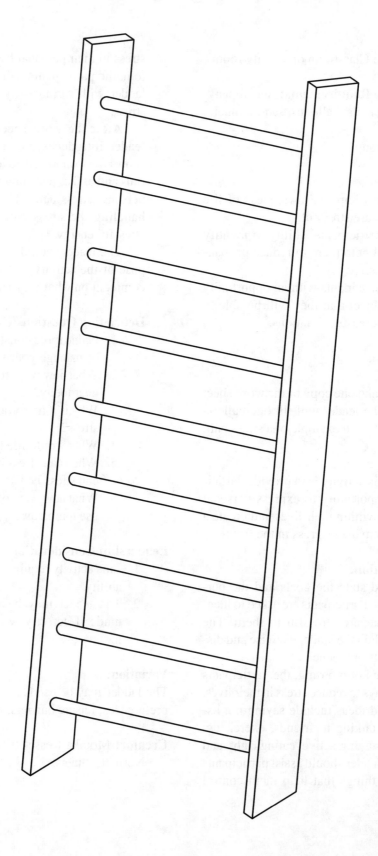

# Positive Physical and
# Mental Health

# My Role Model

**Space Requirements:** Classroom or activity room

**Equipment/Resource Requirements:** Magazines, scissors, glue sticks, paper, writing utensils, role model example

**Group Size:** Small group

**Program Goals:**
1. To increase participants' ability to identify positive characteristics of role models.
2. To increase participants' ability to establish goals of self-improvement.

**Program Description:**
**Preparation:**
The leader should have materials ready before the activity. This includes having an example already assembled and a prepared list of positive qualities a role model might possess for demonstration purposes.

**Introduction:**
The leader will discuss role models and why they are important in everyone's life. Also, the leader and the participants will discuss good and poor qualities to look for in a role model.

**Activity Description:**
The leader distributes the supplies and explains the directions of activity. Each participant will choose a role model from a magazine. After choosing a role model, participants should cut and paste the picture onto their paper. Next, participants should write five positive qualities of the role model that they find admirable.

Then, from the qualities, the participants will write five goals for themselves, stating how they can become more like their role model. The leader will lead a discussion of each person's role model and the goals chosen.

The leader will summarize the activity's goals and purpose and use the following debriefing questions to close the session.

**Debriefing Questions/Closure:**
1. Why is it important to have role models?
2. What is the benefit of having a positive role model?
3. Who would you like to be a role model for?
4. What qualities do you currently possess that would make you a good role model?
5. What actions can you take toward your goals of self-improvement?
6. How realistic are these goals for you?
7. What did you learn from this activity?

**Leadership Considerations:**
1. The leader should assist participants in choosing an appropriate role model.
2. The leader will discuss examples of poor role models and explain why they are poor role models.

**Variations:**
1. The leader may allow participants to choose role models that are directly involved in their lives, i.e., family, teacher, friends.
2. The participants may create their own "ideal" role model, including positive characteristics and traits.

**Creator:** Kristen Boys, Illinois State University, Normal, Illinois.

# Emotion Freeze Tag

**Space Requirements:** Large gymnasium or outside playground grass area

**Equipment/Resource Requirements:** None

**Group Size:** Small or large group

**Program Goals:**
1. To increase participants' awareness of feelings and emotions.
2. To increase participants' awareness of emotional control.
3. To increase participants' awareness of emotional expression.

**Program Description:**
**Preparation:**
The leader will have a discussion ready for introduction. (If possible, the leader should obtain the "emotions poster.")

**Introduction:**
The leader explains to the participants the importance of expressing feelings and emotions. The leader will ask the participants for examples of emotions that they have experienced.

**Activity Description:**
The leader will present the rules of the game: One participant will be designated as the tagger. The other participants then will scatter and the tagger sets out to tag someone. If a participant is being approached to be tagged, he or she must say the name of an emotion or feeling to avoid being tagged. If a participant is unable to do this and he or she is tagged, he or she must freeze and remain in the position in which he or she was tagged until another team member taps him or her on the shoulder and frees him or her. If a participant gets tagged twice, he or she becomes the new tagger.

After playing the game, the participants will sit in a circle for discussion. The leader will lead a discussion on the importance of a balance between emotional control and expression. The leader may use the following debriefing questions for closure.

**Debriefing Questions/Closure:**
1. Was it easy or difficult to come up with different emotions each time you were about to get tagged? Why?
2. Is there any emotion you forgot about using during the game that you can remember now?
3. Why are emotions important?
4. Discuss some situations where you need to control your emotions.
5. What are ways to control your emotions?
6. Discuss some situations where you need to express your emotions.
7. What are ways to express your emotions?
8. What did you learn from this activity?

**Leadership Considerations:**
1. The leader must remember that careful supervision is important considering this is a contact game. The leader will make sure participants do not get out of hand and touch others inappropriately.
2. Giving examples of emotions and feelings may prove helpful to the participants.

**Variation:**
This game originated from freeze tag, and more recently, TV tag. This activity can be used with a variety of skills (e.g., manners, family members, sport heroes).

**Creator:** Kristen Boys, Illinois State University, Normal, Illinois.

# Picture Yourself

**Space Requirements:** Classroom or activity room

**Equipment/Resource Requirements:** Instant camera, film, glue, thick white paper with a square hole cut in the middle (to resemble a picture frame), shape sponges, 8–10 colors of paints

**Group Size:** Small group

**Program Goals:**
1. To increase participants' awareness of positive characteristics of self.
2. To increase participants' awareness of favorable characteristics to acquire.
3. To increase participants' ability to follow directions and remain on task.

**Program Description:**
**Preparation:**
The leader should precut thick paper to resemble a picture frame and set up all other materials prior to starting the activity. The leader should choose ahead of time which traits and characteristics each color of paint will represent. The number of characteristics should be equal to the number of colors of paints. The leader also should make an example to share with the group.

**Introduction:**
The purposes of this activity are for each participant to take notice of the special, positive qualities they possess, and to increase participants' ability to follow directions in order to complete a designated task.

**Activity Description:**
The leader will begin the activity by explaining to the participants that they are going to decorate a picture frame for this activity, but first it will be necessary to have their picture taken. Using an instant camera, the leader will take a picture of each participant. The leader then should set the pictures aside for the time being.

Next, the leader will distribute one blank picture frame to each participant. At this time, the leader will explain to the participants that they will be decorating their picture frame and then putting the picture of themselves into the frame. The leader will explain to the participants that they will not be decorating their frame in just any way; rather, they will decorate it to represent their positive personal characteristics.

The leader will explain that each color of paint will represent a positive trait or characteristic. If individuals feel they possess that trait or characteristic then they can have that color; however, they must first give an example of how they possess that trait or characteristic. For example, if they feel that they are a good friend, they must give reasons to support how they are a good friend. If they do not think they possess that trait or characteristic, then they can state how they can begin practicing that particular trait or characteristic to receive that color.

The leader will encourage participants to be creative in what they paint. They are free to paint their frames however they choose. Once everyone is finished painting his or her picture frame, the leader will give each his or her photo. The photo should be pasted or taped to the backside of the picture frame.

The leader will conclude the activity by having each participant share his or her picture frame with the group. While showing their frame, the participants should discuss the trait or characteristics that most accurately represent them. The leader may close with the following debriefing questions.

**Debriefing Questions/Closure:**
1. Was it easy or difficult to decide what traits you possessed?
2. What did you learn about yourself today?
3. What did you learn about others?
4. What is your most positive feature?
5. What are traits you need to work on?

**Leadership Considerations:**

1. The leader should be supportive and patient with participants. It might take a lot of probing to help them understand the questions and concepts.
2. The leader can provide an example and explain the positive qualities that he or she possesses.
3. Depending on the regulations of the facility, it may be necessary to obtain permission before photographing participants.

**Variations:**

1. The leader may have the participants come up with their own qualities, instead of color-coding them.
2. Instead of simply saying that they have a particular trait or characteristic, the leader may have participants act out how they demonstrate that trait or characteristic, i.e., have the participants show how to be friendly.

**Creator:** Connie Campbell, Illinois State University, Normal, Illinois.

# Feel Good Book

**Space Requirements:** Classroom or activity room

**Equipment/Resource Requirements:** Photo albums, pictures, newspaper clippings, tape, paste, scissors, ribbons, glitter

**Group Size:** Small group

**Program Goal:**
To increase participants' knowledge of positive things or events in their lives.

**Program Description:**
**Preparation:**
The leader will have all supplies ready for the activity session. The leader may have many examples of personal achievements on hand for those participants who are unable to generate ideas.

**Introduction:**
The leader will ask the participants for examples of things that make them smile or bring them joy. The examples can be anything constructive that helps the participants through their day or helps others.

**Activity Description:**
The participants will go through magazines or newspapers for any item or picture that makes them smile or represents something positive—as long as its constructive, it is allowable. The participants will tape or paste these items into their photo albums. The albums represent a variety of positive things that can be used when the participants need a lift.

The leader should encourage the participants to update their books frequently and share them with others. The leader and the participants will discuss the need for focusing on the positive and the benefit of being able to identify things that make them smile or bring them joy.

The leader will close the activity with the following debriefing questions and refocus on the goal of the activity.

**Debriefing Questions/Closure:**
1. How many things have you accomplished in your life that you weren't even aware of?
2. Do you feel better about the type of person you are? Why?
3. Why is it helpful to remember the positive things in your life?
4. Are there certain times when focusing on the positive helps you?
5. What did you learn from this activity that you can use in the future?

**Leadership Considerations:**
1. The leader should have plenty of materials on hand for participants' use. The participants should be allowed to draw or write about what they cannot find.
2. The leader should encourage participants to keep their albums updated.

**Variation:**
The leader may have participants each create a book about who they are. They can include items such as photographs, words, and magazine cutouts.

**Creator:** Kristen Boys, Illinois State University, Normal, Illinois.

# I Can Do

**Space Requirements:** Classroom or activity room

**Equipment/Resource Requirements:** Several sheets of paper (six to eight per participant), scissors, hole puncher, string, stencils, markers or crayons, glue, colored pencils, magazines, stickers

**Program Goals:**
1. To increase participants' awareness of the things they can do that are positive.
2. To increase participants' ability to follow directions in order to complete a designated task.

**Program Description:**
**Preparation:**
The leader will gather supplies and set up the activity area. A completed example should be prepared to share with the group.

**Introduction:**
The purpose of this activity is for the participants to become aware of the positive things that they do and to increase the participants' ability to listen to and follow directions.

**Activity Description:**
The leader will explain to the participants that they are going to make an I Can Do book. The leader will explain and demonstrate directions for constructing the book:

1. Fold the sheets of paper in half (lengthwise).
2. Punch holes on the folded side of the paper.
3. Using the string, tie the pages together.
4. Write the title of the book, *I Can Do,* on the front page. Below the title, write the author's name.
5. Decorate the cover of the book. (The participants should be encouraged to be creative in doing this.)
6. Write a story in the book. The content of the story should reflect what positive things the participants can do, for example, be a good student, be a good friend, be nice to others, be good at a sport.
7. Illustrate the pages of the book. This can be done by drawing pictures or using pictures from magazines.

The participants should be given 30–45 minutes to do this. Once everyone is done, the participants will share their books with the group. The leader will discuss the following debriefing questions.

**Debriefing Questions/Closure:**
1. Name two things that you do really well.
2. How similar or different is this from others in the group?
3. What are you most proud of knowing how to do?
4. How can you put this to good use?
5. How can being more aware of things you do well help you?
6. What did you learn about yourself today?

**Leadership Considerations:**
1. Constant support and encouragement will be needed to help participants come up with things that they can do.
2. The leader should be aware of the cognitive level of the group.
3. The leader should be ready to assist in writing "I Can Do" statements in participants' books.

**Variations:**
1. The leader may alter the content of the book, i.e., use compliments.
2. This book may be used for community and/ or home resources.

**Creator:** Connie Campbell, Illinois State University, Normal, Illinois.

# Differences Can Be Positive

**Space Requirements:** Classroom or activity room; outdoor area

**Equipment/Resource Requirements:** Drawing paper, markers and crayons, leaves collected from outside, chalkboard or dry erase board, chalk or markers

**Group Size:** Small group

**Program Goals:**
1. To increase participants' ability to identify differences among individuals in the group.
2. To improve participants' understanding of the positives that can result from these differences.
3. To increase participants' ability to follow directions.

**Program Description:**
**Preparation:**
The leader will gather the necessary supplies.

**Introduction:**
The purpose of the activity is to improve participants' ability to identify differences among individuals and to increase their ability to identify the positives that can result from being different.

**Activity Description:**
The leader will introduce the activity by explaining that the activity focuses on differences in individuals and how differences are not always negative. Prior to beginning the outdoor portion of the activity, the leader will inform the participants that he or she will be taking them outside. The leader will explain that once they get outside, the participants will be responsible for collecting three to five different types of leaves.

The leader will take the group outside and allow approximately 10 minutes to collect leaves, ensuring that all individuals of the group stay within sight of the staff. Once all individuals have collected three to five leaves, the group will return to the activity room.

Upon returning, the leader will instruct the participants to set aside their leaves. At this point, the leader will list each group member's name on the board (vertically). Next, the leader will ask each individual to identify his or her hair color, eye color, and skin color. As the participants respond, the leader will write their answers on the board, below each name. Once all participants have their information listed on the board, the leader will distribute three sheets of paper to each person in the group.

The participants will outline both of their hands on the first page. Next they will outline both of their feet on the second page. When the participants have completed the tracing of their hands and feet, they will arrange their leaves on the table so that the third sheet of paper will completely cover the leaves.

When the leaves and paper are in place, the leader will give each of the participants one crayon and instruct them to take the paper off the crayon. Next, the leader will tell them to rub the crayon on top of the paper, from side to side, top to bottom. By following these directions, the outline of the leaves should appear on the page.

When all group members have completed the leaf rubbings, the leader should collect all three drawings from each person and place all of the hands in one row, all of the feet in one row, and all of the leaf rubbings in one row. The participants are asked to identify the similarities and differences between all of the drawings as well as the information on the board. The leader may want to focus on each area individually (for example, discuss the board first, hands second, feet third, and leaves fourth). The leader will close the activity with the following debriefing questions.

**Debriefing Questions/Closure:**

1. Identify the similarities among the individuals in the group; that is, about the similarities among the hands, feet, and leaves. Identify the differences.
2. How might an individual identify or treat these differences as negative?
3. How can the differences identified be positive?
4. What are some ways you can focus on the positive of these differences rather than the negative?
5. How will you use this information today and tomorrow?

**Leadership Considerations:**

1. The leader should inform the participants that the outline of the feet can be done with or without shoes on.
2. The leader may want to discuss each part of the activity as it is completed rather than processing all parts at the end of the activity.

3. The leader may want to have examples of leaf rubbings prepared prior to the start of the activity to use as an example.
4. Some participants may need assistance when tracing hands and feet.

**Variations:**

1. The leader may divide the group into teams and see which team can identify the most differences and the most positive aspects of those differences.
2. The leader may ask participants to identify personal character traits that are unique to them and then lead a discussion on how these characteristics are different and also discuss how these differences can be positive.
3. Participants may create a list of positives that can come from being different, and the leader can make the list available for all participants to keep.

**Creator:** Theresa M. Connolly, CTRS, Illinois State University, Normal, Illinois.

# Grab Bag Relay

**Space Requirements:** Gymnasium or large activity room

**Equipment/Resource Requirements:** List of Grab Bag activities (two copies), timer or stopwatch, paper grocery bag, basketball, jump rope, soccer ball, two balloons, two sticks of gum, four saltine crackers

**Group Size:** Small group

**Program Goals:**
1. To increase participants' awareness of self-strengths.
2. To improve participants' problem-solving skills.
3. To improve participants' ability to follow directions.

**Program Description:**
**Preparation:**
Depending on the number of participants in the group, the leader will develop a list of Grab Bag activities that would enable each participant to "grab" a minimum of two or three activities. The leader will cut up one copy of the list into separate slips of paper, fold the slips of paper, and place them into the paper grocery bag. Examples of activities include:

- Run the perimeter of the gym and return to your group;
- While lying on your back, count backward from 25 to 0;
- Rub your belly, pat your head, while spinning in a circle 5 times;
- Sing "Mary Had a Little Lamb;"
- Jump like a frog and say, "Ribbit," back to your group;
- Do 5 somersaults;
- Do 5 cartwheels;
- Do 15 sit-ups;
- Do 5 push-ups;

- Run, while jumping rope, to the opposite end of the gym and return to your group;
- Dribble the soccer ball (with your feet) to the far end of the gym and back;
- Jump rope in place 10 times in a row; start over if you miss one;
- Shoot a free throw;
- Shoot the basketball from the 3-point line;
- Sing the alphabet song out loud;
- With your eyes closed, spin around 10 times then run back to your group;
- Do 15 jumping jacks;
- Do a handstand and see how long you can stay in the air;
- Blow up the balloon, tie it, and pop it by sitting on it;
- Chew the piece of gum and then blow a bubble; and
- Eat two saltine crackers, then whistle.

One balloon, one stick of gum, and two saltine crackers should be placed in the grocery bag with the activity slips. All other necessary equipment (soccer ball, jump rope, basketball) will be placed near the grocery bag.

**Introduction:**
The leader will explain to the participants that they will be playing a relay game which will require them to work together as a team, and they are to give positive support to one another.

**Activity Description:**
The participants will line up behind a line 15 feet away from the grocery bag. The leader will inform the participants that only one person may go at a time. Each person must run to the bag, draw a slip of paper from the bag, read the message on the slip of paper aloud, and then perform the activity described on the paper. When the activity has been completed, the participant must

run back to the group and the next participant will repeat the process. If a participant is unable to perform the task, the participant may place the slip back into the bag and draw a new activity.

The leader, using the stopwatch, should keep track of the amount of time it takes for the participants to complete all of the activities.

When the participants have completed the activity, the leader will explain that they will repeat the relay, but this time they may choose who will complete each task. The leader will give the second copy of the activity list to the group and give the participants 5 to 10 minutes to problem solve as a group and to assign tasks to each participant. All participants must be assigned an equal number of activities, and the activities should be assigned according to the strengths of each participant.

The participants will complete the relay a second time. Again, the leader will keep track of the amount of time it takes to complete the relay the second time. When all of the activities have been completed, the participants will compare times to see if the second relay took a longer or shorter period of time to complete.

The leader will refocus on the goals and discuss the following questions.

**Debriefing Questions/Closure:**
1. Explain what happened the first time you completed the relay.
2. How was the second time different?
3. What process did you use to solve the problem of assigning each activity to each team member?
4. What was difficult about acknowledging your self-strengths, if anything?
5. How did it feel to have others recognize your strengths?
6. Why is it important to point out the positives in others?
7. How does everyone's strengths help move a team forward?

**Leadership Considerations:**
1. If a participant is unable to read, the leader or another participant may read the slips.
2. The leader should encourage participants to cheer for one another throughout the relay.
3. The leader should encourage participants to complete a task even if they feel unable to do so.

**Variations:**
1. Rather than keeping the rest of the group standing still until their turn comes along, the leader may have each participant draw a slip, read the slip to the group, and then have the entire group complete each task together.
2. The leader may divide the group into two teams and have the teams compete against one another.
3. The leader may alter the content of the activities on the list to include the expression of emotions to group members (i.e., name three ways to control anger; say one positive comment about each teammate).

**Creator:** Theresa M. Connolly, CTRS, Illinois State University, Normal, Illinois.

# Everything I Ever Wanted to Do But Didn't . . . Because I Was Afraid

**Space Requirements:** Classroom or activity room

**Equipment/Resource Requirements:** Accompanying form, chalkboard or large drawing paper, pencils, additional drawing paper, markers, crayons, colored pencils

**Group Size:** Small group

**Program Goals:**
1. To increase participants' ability to acknowledge activities they want to do, but never have.
2. To increase participants' ability to identify personal fears.
3. To improve participants' ability to identify ways to overcome fears.

**Program Description:**
**Preparation:**
The leader should have all materials prepared prior to the start of the activity.

**Introduction:**
The purpose of this activity is to encourage participants to identify activities that they desire to participate in and any fears that keep them from participating.

**Activity Description:**
The leader will introduce the activity and explain that it will deal with everything the participants have ever wanted to do but didn't because they were afraid. As a group, the leader and participants will review the checklist. Then the participants will be asked to identify activities in which they wish to participate. The leader should write these activities on the chalkboard or large drawing paper for all of the group to see.

Once participants have completed the list, each person will identify the fears that most typically represent why the desired activities were not carried out. After this step is completed, the leader will distribute drawing materials and ask participants to draw a picture of what they imagine fear to look like and what represents fear in their lives.

When the drawings are complete, the participants will write all fears (those listed and not listed) on the same page as the drawing. Once all drawings are completed, the leader and participants will discuss as a group each of the drawings using the following closure questions.

**Debriefing Questions/Closure:**
1. Name some of the activities you've wanted to do.
2. What are some of the fears you have in relation to the activities you'd like to do?
3. Do any of these fears also appear on your drawing?
4. How can you overcome or cope with your fears?
5. Name one thing you learned about yourself from completing this activity.

**Leadership Considerations:**
1. The participants should be given plenty of time to complete the checklist.
2. The leader may make a list of suggested ways to cope with fears and distribute a copy to each participant.
3. The leader should encourage participants to give feedback to peers.
4. The leader may allow participants to use drawings rather than words.

**Variations:**
1. The participants could work together to do a group drawing of fear.
2. The participants could create a list of coping skills or strategies to overcome fears.
3. List of wants could be changed to things the participants have already done that have made them feel those fears.

**Creator:** Theresa M. Connolly, CTRS, Illinois State University, Normal, Illinois.

# Everything I Ever Wanted to Do But Didn't . . . Because I Was Afraid

| Everything I Ever Wanted to Do: | Fears: I'll fail | Feel stupid | Feel unattractive | Unsure of self | Hurt by another | Not be liked | Feel guilty | Lose everything | Others get mad at me | Lose job | Something bad will happen to me | Couldn't live with self | Other |
|---|---|---|---|---|---|---|---|---|---|---|---|---|---|
| 1. | | | | | | | | | | | | | |
| 2. | | | | | | | | | | | | | |
| 3. | | | | | | | | | | | | | |
| 4. | | | | | | | | | | | | | |
| 5. | | | | | | | | | | | | | |
| 6. | | | | | | | | | | | | | |
| 7. | | | | | | | | | | | | | |
| 8. | | | | | | | | | | | | | |
| 9. | | | | | | | | | | | | | |
| 10. | | | | | | | | | | | | | |
| 11. | | | | | | | | | | | | | |
| 12. | | | | | | | | | | | | | |
| 13. | | | | | | | | | | | | | |
| 14. | | | | | | | | | | | | | |
| 15. | | | | | | | | | | | | | |
| 16. | | | | | | | | | | | | | |
| 17. | | | | | | | | | | | | | |
| 18. | | | | | | | | | | | | | |
| 19. | | | | | | | | | | | | | |
| 20. | | | | | | | | | | | | | |

# All About You and Me

**Space Requirements:** Classroom or activity room

**Equipment/Resource Requirements:** Pens, pencils, crayons, markers, paper

**Group Size:** Small group

**Program Goals:**
1. To increase participants' awareness of activities they enjoy.
2. To increase participants' ability to identify positive self qualities.

**Program Description:**
**Preparation:**
The leader will place all needed supplies on the table or working area. He or she may want to draw a picture of himself or herself and list three things about himself or herself. This then can be used as an example for the group to help the participants feel more comfortable about the activity.

**Introduction:**
The purpose of this activity is to heighten participants' self-awareness, and allow them the opportunity to exercise appropriate and positive social and communication skills.

To begin the activity, the leader will initiate a discussion on getting to know one another. A suggestion for a discussion is as follows:

In order for us to feel more comfortable as a group, it is important to get to know one another. This activity will help us each identify something we like to do and at least three positive qualities we have.

**Activity Description:**
The leader will begin the activity by passing a piece of paper, pens, pencils, markers and crayons to each participant. The leader then will explain to the participants that they are to close their eyes and picture themselves doing an activity they enjoy. Once they get a vision in their head, they then are to draw this on the piece of paper. After participants complete their drawings, they should each write down three positive qualities that they possess.

The leader then will begin a discussion about the pictures that the participants have drawn and ask them to talk about their positive qualities. To make the discussion less intimidating, the leader may begin by talking about the picture he or she drew and the things he or she wrote. After each participant has shared a minimum of one quality from his or her drawing the leader will ask the following debriefing questions.

**Debriefing Questions/Closure:**
1. How did you choose the qualities you did?
2. Would others agree these are positive qualities you have?
3. How did it feel to draw yourself in a situation you enjoy?
4. How did it feel to share positive things about yourself with the rest of the group?
5. What are some benefits of knowing your positive qualities?

**Leadership Considerations:**
1. The leader should not force the participants to share their answers. It should be their choice of how much information they want to disclose.
2. The participants should be given time to think of a situation they enjoy. They should not be rushed.

**Variations:**
1. Each participant may draw a picture frame around the paper and frame his or her work.
2. Instead of visualizing an activity they enjoy doing, the participants could draw a self-portrait.

3. The participants may do all the same steps, but when they are done with their drawing and positive qualities, the leader will divide them into pairs and have them tell the other person about who they are. Then, the other person tells the group about the person he or she interviewed.

**Creator:** Amy Conron, Illinois State University, Normal, Illinois.

# Express Yourself

**Space Requirements:** Classroom or activity room

**Equipment/Resource Requirements:** Large sheets of white construction paper (one per participant), various colors of glitter, glue, tempera paints, letter-shaped sponges, markers, newspaper

**Group Size:** Small group

**Program Goal:**
To increase participants' awareness of positive characteristics of self.

**Program Description:**
**Preparation:**
The leader should have a completed example to share with the group. Newspapers should be spread out on top of tables.

**Introduction:**
The purpose of this activity is to give participants the opportunity to creatively express favorable leisure activities and positive characteristics of self. Prior to explaining directions of activity, it may be necessary for the leader to discuss and provide examples of leisure activities and positive self characteristics.

**Activity Description:**
The leader will distribute one piece of paper to each participant and explain directions: The first step is for the participant to put his or her name in the center of the paper. This can be done in one of two ways:

1. Squeezing the bottle of glue, spell out the name (in large letters), then sprinkle glitter on top of the glue. Shake excess glitter off onto newspaper and replace in glitter container.
2. Dip the letter-shaped sponges into paint and then apply to center of paper.

The next step is for the participants to add to their picture by responding to the following sentences:

1. My best skill is _____.
2. My best personality characteristic is _____.
3. People like me because _____.
4. The part of my body I like most is _____.
5. I'm a good friend because _____.

The leader should encourage the participants to be creative in doing this step. Last, the participants may finish decorating their artwork in anyway they choose. Once everyone is finished, each participant will explain his or her picture to the group. The leader will conclude the activity by discussing the following questions.

**Debriefing Questions/Closure:**
1. Can you think of additional things to include on your picture about yourself?
2. Was it easy or difficult to think of a positive characteristic of yourself?
3. Why is it important to recognize what we do well?
4. What did you learn about others in the group?

**Leadership Considerations:**
1. The leader should encourage participants to be creative.
2. The leader should offer praise when the participants are trying to complete the task.
3. The leader can give the participants ideas of what they can put on their sheet.

**Variation:**
The leader may allow the participants to paste cutout pictures from magazines on their pictures.

**Creator:** Connie Campbell, Illinois State University, Normal, Illinois.

# Stars

**Space Requirements:** Classroom or activity room

**Equipment/Resource Requirements:** Scissors, paper, markers and/or crayons

**Group Size:** Small group

**Program Goals:**
1. To increase participants' awareness of positive qualities of self.
2. To improve participants' awareness of personal needs.

**Program Description:**
**Preparation:**
Prior to implementing the activity, the leader will need to outline one large star on each sheet of paper. The participants will each cut a star out during the activity. On one side of the star, the phrase, "I am a star," should be written. On the other side, the phrase, "I wish upon a star," should be written. Either the leader can do this ahead of time or the participants may do this themselves.

**Introduction:**
This activity is designed to help individuals realize not only their positive qualities, but also their potential. It also can be used as a tool to improve self-awareness.

**Activity Description:**
Each participant will be given a piece of paper with a large star shape drawn on it. Participants will be instructed to cut out the star shape. On one side of the star will be the phrase, "I am a star," on the other side will be the phrase, "I wish upon a star." The participants will be instructed to draw pictures of all of the things they are good at on the side labeled "I am a star."

Once this step is completed they will turn the star over to the side labeled "I wish upon a star." On this side they will draw or write quali-

ties that they want to acquire or become better at. Examples could include being a good friend, a good student, or polite.

When all stars are completed, the group members will get into a circle and discuss all of their good qualities. Next, the group members will discuss the qualities they wish to have or improve upon and how that can happen. The leader will refocus on the goals of the activity and close the activity with the following discussion questions.

**Debriefing Questions/Closure:**
1. What qualities do you have that make you a star? Why?
2. What qualities do you wish to have that you do not already have?
3. What qualities do you wish to improve upon?
4. How can you go about obtaining these positive qualities?
5. What are the benefits of recognizing your own personal qualities?
6. What are the benefits of identifying areas where you'd like to improve?

**Leadership Considerations:**
1. The leader may have an example prepared to show participants what is expected of them.
2. The leader may give examples of various positive qualities to initiate the participants' thoughts about themselves.

**Variation:**
Participants could make a mobile by attaching strings to numerous stars and then hanging them from a coat hanger. The participants could write down different ways that they could gain new, additional positive qualities on the stars.

**Creator:** Jessica Kamm, Illinois State University, Normal, Illinois.

# Personal Cereal

**Space Requirements:** Classroom or activity room

**Equipment/Resource Requirements:** Markers, paper, glue, empty cereal boxes

**Group Size:** Small group

**Program Goals:**
1. To improve participants' ability to identify positive personal qualities.
2. To increase participants' self-awareness.

**Program Description:**
**Preparation:**
The leader will gather supplies and have a completed example to share with the group.

**Introduction:**
The purpose of this activity is to improve the participants' ability to identify positive personal qualities and improve their self-awareness. The leader will explain to the participants that they will design and decorate their own cereal box in a creative way.

**Activity Description:**
Each participant will receive his or her own supplies (markers, paper, glue and one empty cereal box). Once the participants receive the materials, they can begin to assemble a personal cereal box. This process begins by first covering an empty cereal box with the blank paper. The next step is to create a cereal name that represents him or her (e.g., Special J for a participant named Jim).

After a name is chosen, participants are to design a logo that expresses their positive qualities. Last, the participants will write a list of ingredients contained in the cereal. The ingredients should reflect each of their unique personal qualities (e.g., an ounce of caring, a cup of trustworthiness).

The activity will conclude with a discussion of the meaning of each of the cereal boxes. The group will discuss the following debriefing questions to close the activity.

**Debriefing Questions/Closure:**
1. Why did you choose the name of the cereal that you chose?
2. Explain why or how it represents you.
3. What kinds of ingredients have you included in your cereal?
4. Give some examples showing these qualities at school.
5. How do your ingredients differ from others in the group?
6. How can you put your ingredients to good use?
7. What makes your cereal (you) unique?

**Leadership Considerations:**
1. The leader may have a cereal box prepared to use as an example for the group.
2. The leader may give examples of different qualities that participants might possess.
3. The leader should encourage all individuals to have at least seven ingredients.

**Variation:**
Instead of creating a cereal name and cereal boxes, the participants may write an advertisement for a toy doll. They should give the toy doll the characteristics of themselves.

**Creator:** Jessica Kamm, Illinois State University, Normal, Illinois.

# Value Expressions

**Space Requirements:** Classroom or activity room

**Equipment/Resource Requirements:** Thick construction paper, paintbrushes, tempera (washable) paint

**Group Size:** Small group

**Program Goals:**
1. To increase participants' understanding of the importance of having values.
2. To increase participants' recognition of what they value most in life.

**Program Description:**
**Preparation:**
The leader will prepare completed examples to share with the group.

**Introduction:**
The purpose of this activity is to have participants understand their own values and the importance of values. The leader will explain to participants that they will be doing an art activity about personal values.

**Activity Description:**
The leader will begin the activity by initiating a discussion on what values are, why they are important to have, and why it is important to express or demonstrate to others what one's values are. After a general discussion of values, each participant will choose (from a list if necessary) one to three values that are most important to him or her. Then, the participants will brainstorm different ways to express those particular values. The leader should be prepared to give an example.

Following the discussion, the leader will explain that art (specifically painting) is a good way of expressing values without using verbal expression. The leader will explain that is what the par-

ticipants will be doing during this activity. Next, the leader will distribute the supplies and have each participant paint a picture of one value he or she considers to be very important. This picture should represent a situation that demonstrates that he or she holds this particular value.

Once everyone has completed his or her painting, the participants will try and guess what value is represented in each other's picture. If time allows, the participants may choose another value they think they possess and repeat the process. The finished paintings may be displayed underneath the heading "What We Value" and placed in a public area for everyone to see.

The leader will close the activity by refocusing on the goals of the activity.

**Debriefing Questions/Closure:**
1. How do we benefit from having values?
2. How do values affect behavior?
3. How does expressing values in a positive way show what one believes in?
4. Have you ever thought about your values before doing this activity?
5. How can you tell what someone's values are?
6. What values would you like to acquire or improve upon?

**Leadership Consideration:**
A higher cognitive level is needed to participate in this activity.

**Variations:**
1. The participants may paint a picture of the characteristics they look for in a friend.
2. The participants may paint a picture of a situation they were in where they exercised a value.

**Creator:** Sandra Larson, Illinois State University, Normal, Illinois.

# Obstacle of Values

**Space Requirements:** Large activity room, gymnasium or outside area

**Equipment/Resource Requirements:** Various sporting equipment, balloons, note cards

**Group Size:** Small group

**Program Goals:**
1. To increase participants' awareness of personal values exercised.
2. To allow participants the opportunity to engage in quick and efficient decision-making skills.
3. To allow participants the opportunity to engage in physical activity.

**Program Description:**
**Preparation:**
The leader will set up an obstacle course (preferably in a large gym). Each station will represent a different task that needs to be completed (e.g., dribbling a basketball around cones, doing 10 jumping jacks). Also, the leader will place questions at each station for the participants to answer before moving on to the next station (see accompanying list for examples). The questions should deal with values.

**Introduction:**
The leader will explain to the group members that they will be involved in an obstacle course activity. They will go to each station, do the required activity, and answer a question. At this point, the leader will guide the entire group through the obstacle course and show the participants what each station represents, and what activity they will be required to do.

**Activity Description:**
The participants line up at the start area. The leader will explain to the group members that they will each take a turn completing the obstacle course. The leader will accompany each person to each station and keep track of the amount of time it takes each person to go through the entire course. The leader may either ask for volunteers to go first or use a systematic way of beginning.

As the leader accompanies each person, he or she will be the judge of determining if a participant answers a question correctly. If a question is not answered correctly, the leader will add 15 seconds to that person's finishing time.

After each participant has had a minimum of one turn, the leader will hold a discussion on the importance of having values. The participants will sit in a circle and discuss the following debriefing questions.

**Debriefing Questions/Closure:**
1. What are examples of values?
2. How are values displayed?
3. Have you ever given serious consideration to what your values are?
4. How are other people's values sometimes different than your own?
5. Why is it important to be aware of your values?

**Leadership Considerations:**
1. The leader should make sure each person is able to do the physical aspect of the activity.
2. The leader should make sure all equipment and stations are set up safely.
3. The leader may want to have another individual assist in supervising the participants while they are waiting to go through the obstacle course.

**Variation:**
The leader may use different content areas for the questions.

**Creator:** Sandra Larson, Illinois State University, Normal, Illinois.

# Obstacle of Values

## Sample Question List

1. If a world without lying and cheating is important to me, I value:
   a. Good health
   b. Honesty
   c. Wisdom

2. I value Justice because . . .
   a. Fairness is important to me
   b. School is important to me
   c. Eating is important to me

3. Approval from others is important to me.
   a. True
   b. False

4. I value Friendships because . . .
   a. Good grades are important to me
   b. Playing games is important to me
   c. Social relationships are important to me

5. I would exercise and eat healthy foods if I value . . .
   a. Emotional well-being
   b. Achievement
   c. Good health

6. I finish tasks I start because I value . . .
   a. Achievement
   b. Justice
   c. Love

7. I value Knowledge because I . . .
   a. Always brush my teeth before bed time
   b. Tell the truth most of the time
   c. Try to pay attention and learn in school

8. Having self-confidence is important to me, so I must value . . .
   a. Recognition
   b. Emotional well-being
   c. Pleasure

9. One way to show Honesty is to . . .
   a. Watch a lot of television
   b. Tell the truth
   c. Not answer people's questions

# All About Me

**Space Requirements:** Classroom or activity room

**Equipment/Resource Requirements:** One large sheet of paper per participant (long and wide enough to trace a body on), Magic Markers (washable)

**Group Size:** Small group

**Program Goals:**
1. To increase participants' self-awareness.
2. To increase participants' awareness of what makes an individual unique.
3. To increase participants' ability to follow directions and remain on task.

**Program Description:**
**Preparation:**
The leader should prepare a completed example to share with the group.

**Introduction:**
The leader will explain to the participants that everyone is made up of different traits and that is what makes each person unique. The leader and participants will discuss some of those traits that make each person unique.

**Activity Description:**
The leader will distribute one piece of paper to each participant and place markers in an area within reach of all group members. Participants will be paired into groups of two. Each participant will trace his or her partner's body onto the piece of paper with a marker. The leader will instruct participants to be careful not to mark their partner's clothes with the markers.

Next, each participant will find an area on the table or floor to spread his or her body tracing on. At this time the participants will cut out the tracing of their body. Once this is done, the leader will instruct each person to get a marker

and get ready to follow the directions. The directions are to be read by the leader:

1. Show on your head what you want to be when you grow up.
2. Show on your mouth what the name of your favorite song is.
3. Show on your hands what you like to do best with your hands.
4. Show on your heart which person you would love to be or which person you admire most.
5. Show your favorite food on your stomach.
6. Show on your thigh where your dream vacation spot is.
7. Show on your foot what sport or activity you like to do best.

While answering these questions, participants can begin by simply writing the answer, and then if time allows, they can draw a picture to represent the answer they have written.

The leader will conclude the activity by having each participant answer the following questions while showing his or her body tracing to the group. Following the discussion, the participants may hang their body tracing on a wall in the facility. The leader should reemphasize how everyone is special and unique.

**Debriefing Questions/Closure:**
1. What is the most unique feature about you?
2. Why is it important to be unique in some ways?
3. What are some similarities and differences between group members?
4. What is one way you're different from everyone else here?
5. What is one difference that you are really proud of?

**Leadership Considerations:**
1. If the participants are unable to write, the leader should allow more time for them to draw their answers.
2. Participants should spread out around the room when drawing so that they don't distract others.
3. The leader should be aware of participants who may have an issue about their body image.

**Variations:**
1. The content of what is correlated with body parts may be changed to meet the needs of the participants.
2. The participants may make up the questions to be answered on their body tracing.

**Creator:** Amanda L. McGowen, Illinois State University, Normal, Illinois.

# Responsibility in the Classroom

**Space Requirements:** Gymnasium or large activity room

**Equipment/Resource Requirements:** Discussion and game note cards, tray, small items (to put on tray for the first activity), paper, writing utensils

**Group Size:** Small group

**Program Goals:**
1. To exercise participants' short-term memory recall skills.
2. To increase participants' awareness of rules and responsibilities in a classroom.

**Program Description:**
**Preparation:**
The leader will prepare the game note cards and place a variety of different, small items on a tray (no more than twenty). Pieces of yarn, money, toothpicks, buttons, thread, jewelry, and pencils are all good examples of the kinds of things to put on this tray.

**Introduction:**
The leader will cover the tray with a piece of cloth so participants cannot see what is on the tray. The tray should be placed in an area where everyone can gather around to see what's on it when it's time. The leader will give each participant a piece of paper and a writing utensil.

**Activity Description:**
*Part 1:*
The leader will explain to the participants that they will have two minutes to study the objects on the tray once it is uncovered. After the two minutes are up, the leader will take the tray away. At this time, the participants must write on their piece of paper what items were on the tray. The leader will allow two minutes for this.

The leader will set ground rules: The participants can't talk to each other or other groups (un-less they are working in pairs), and no one is al-lowed to sneak preview the materials on the tray or look at the tray after it has been re-covered.

After two minutes, everyone will be re-minded to put their pencils down. The leader will find out how many items each person could re-member by telling the group all of the items that were on the tray.

At this time, the leader will explain to the participants that they will now be doing Part 2 of this activity. Part 2 will require them to exercise their memory again.

*Part 2:*
The leader will give each participant a note card. The note card will have a number on one side and a question on the other (see the accompany-ing Part 2 questions). The leader will instruct the participants to line up in numerical order accord-ing to the number on their cards. Next, remain-ing in the same line up, the group will form a circle and sit on the floor. At this time the par-ticipants will read the statements on their cards and discuss the answers.

The leader will explain that it may be diffi-cult to remember the rules sometimes just like it was hard to remember all the items on the tray. The leader may say, "It is good to review the rules to yourself often so that you can remember them easily."

*Part 3:*
The setting for this part of the activity should be a gymnasium or large activity area. The game is a version of freeze tag. The leader will ask ev-eryone to line up at one end of the gym. The leader will stand directly in the center of the gym.

To play the game, the leader will call out a color. Everyone wearing that color will attempt to run across the gym. When the leader calls, "Freeze," all the people running need to freeze. The last one to freeze has to answer a question (see the accompanying Part 3 questions).

If participants answer incorrectly, they must sit down in the spot where they froze. While they are sitting they should try to tag someone out who is running by them. However, they are required to remain on the floor while doing this. If the participants answer the question correctly, they may remain standing and continue across the gym when their color is called again.

When all the questions have been used a minimum of one time or when time is up, the game will end. The participants will sit in a circle and discuss the following debriefing questions.

**Debriefing Questions/Closure:**
1. What is an example of a rule used in the classroom?
2. For what occasions do you have to follow rules?
3. It can sometimes be difficult to remember all the rules all of the time, but if you practice and remind yourself of them it will likely get easier. What are ways you can practice remembering rules?

4. What are the consequences if you do not follow rules? What are the consequences if none of us followed the rules?

**Leadership Considerations:**
1. The leader should make sure that all participants are able to read and write.
2. It may be necessary to have a discussion on what responsibility is and give several examples before playing Part 2 of the activity.
3. The leader should allow plenty of time so that all three parts of the activity can be fully completed.

**Variation:**
At the end of the activity, the participants may play the memory game as they did in the beginning. The leader will have the participants compare how many more they remembered than the last time. It helps to review and practice!

**Creator:** Amanda L. McGowen, Illinois State University, Normal, Illinois.

# Responsibility in the Classroom

## Part 2 Questions

1. Why do think there are rules like "No talking when the teacher is talking"?
2. What if your best friend was sitting right behind you in class and you had something really important to tell him or her? Should you talk then?
3. Why might it bother other people if you were talking?
4. What are some times during the school day when you could talk to your friends?
5. When a teacher asks you to do something, what do you usually do?
6. Why do you think students put off doing things that the teacher asks them to do?
7. What does the teacher expect you to do when he or she asks you to do something?
8. What would it sound like in a room if everyone talked at once?
9. What are some things at school that should be done with everyone being quiet?
10. What are some things at school that can be done without being quiet?
11. What are some clues that you may see that let you know it is time to quiet down?

# Responsibility in the Classroom

## Part 3 Questions

*Category 1:* Talking to your neighbor. Is this a good time to be talking to him or her: yes or no?

1. The teacher is telling the answers to your science quiz. You got a lot of them wrong and want to ask your friend what answers she had. Is this a good time to ask her? Why?
2. You are in art class and the teacher is explaining how to mix the paints properly. You already know how to do this and want to tell your neighbor all about the movie you saw last night. Is this a good time to tell him? Why?
3. It's lunchtime and you are sitting by your friends. You want to tell them about what you want to do this upcoming weekend. Is this a good time to tell them? Why?
4. You just got dismissed from school for the day and you want to tell your friend about all the birthday presents you got over the weekend. Is this a good time? Why?
5. It's a tornado drill and while you are lining up you want to tell your friend how you saw the movie *Twister.* Is this a good time? Why?
6. All of your work is finished for the day, so the teacher lets you go to the back table and work on an art project with a friend. You have a great idea for a picture and want to ask your partner what she thinks. Is this a good time? Why?

*Category 2:* Following the teacher's instructions. Is the student doing what the teacher asked him or her to do right away: yes or no?

1. Mrs. Tames asked Joan to put her pencil down. She put it in her ear. Is Joan doing what the teacher asked?
2. Ms. Morgan asked the class to line up at the door. Alex began to go over and sharpen his pencil. Was Alex doing what the teacher asked?
3. Mrs. Wilkins asked Steve to put away his markers. Steve continued to color on his sheet of paper. Is Steve doing what the teacher asked?
4. Mr. Stein asked Kay to come up to the blackboard. Kay walked over to her desk. Is Kay doing what the teacher asked her to do?
5. Mr. Jones asked Jason to take a note to the principal's office. He took it straight there. Is he doing what the teacher asked him to do?

*Category 3:* Knowing the best times to quiet down. Answer yes or no to each situation if you think it is a good time for the class to quiet down.

1. The last bell has rang and it's time to go home.
2. The teacher is giving instructions on what to bring the next day for the field trip.
3. It is recess time and everyone is outside.
4. The bell for the fire drill just went off.
5. A guest just walked into the room to teach you about interesting animals.
6. The teacher is getting ready to teach the class how to use a new computer in the classroom.
7. The art teacher is explaining how to make modeling clay.
8. The teacher is explaining that if everyone works quickly the whole class can go outside for free time.

# Recognizing Personality Differences in People

**Space Requirements:** Classroom or activity room

**Equipment/Resource Requirements:** Magazines, two pieces of poster board, glue, scissors

**Group Size:** Small group

**Program Goal:**
To increase participants' ability to identify descriptive characteristics of their peers.

**Program Description:**
**Preparation:**
The leader will gather the supplies including a variety of magazines for participants to look through. These will be used to find different personality traits. It will be beneficial for the participants if there is an example of a personality poster for them to see ahead of time.

**Introduction:**
The leader will begin the activity by explaining that sometimes when one describes a person, the first characteristic mentioned is not what the person looks like or where he or she goes to play:

> If I asked you to describe a clown, what would you say? (Silly) Or if I asked you to describe someone who helped you up after you fell down, what would you say? (Very nice)

These are characteristics of a person's personality, what he or she is like on the inside.

The participants should list as many personality characteristics as they can in one minute. Examples of personality characteristics include generous, bossy, kind, happy, selfish, friendly, loud, shy, and outgoing. The leader can write these on a chalkboard if he or she chooses.

**Activity Description:**
The leader will divide the participants into two groups. The leader will explain that the group members are going to be working as a team to decide the best word to describe the people who they will hear a little about. Each team will have about 30 seconds to come up with a decision.

They will have a list of words from which to choose. After the description is read each team will have the opportunity to share the descriptive word the team members agreed on. Each person on each team should be given the opportunity to share the word in front of the group.

If the team(s) guesses the correct descriptive word, the team wins a point. The team with the most points wins. It may be necessary to have an adult in each group to help facilitate a positive team-working environment.

These are the words that each group will need to have available either written on a piece of paper or on a chalkboard that is visible:

- friendly,
- helpful,
- loud,
- mean,
- selfish, and
- shy.

The following descriptions are to be read to the participants (answers are in parentheses):

1. Ronald never shares his toys with anyone. He grabs them away from other people and says, "MINE!" (Selfish)
2. Sally talks to new kids when they come into the class and do not know anyone. She knows it's hard to be new and not have any friends. (Friendly)
3. David doesn't like to meet new people. He looks down at the floor and doesn't say anything. (Shy)

4. Claudia pulls other people's hair and makes them mad. She runs away laughing. (Mean)
5. Sam notices that a little girl can't reach the toys on the top shelf. He helped her reach the toys. (Helpful)
6. Mike is always yelling, even when he isn't mad at anybody. "Quiet down!" the teacher is always telling him. "Shhhhhhh!" (Loud)

The leader should congratulate each team on a job well done. The participants will stay in the same teams while the leader explains that each team is going to make a characteristic poster. The participants will compile pictures of faces (from magazines) expressing different characteristics and combine them into one poster for each team.

When each team has completed its poster, the team members will share it with the larger group and describe the pictures they have included on it. The activity concludes with discussion of the following questions.

**Debriefing Questions/Closure:**
1. Name three personality characteristics represented on the posters.

2. How does a person's personality show up in his or her behavior?
3. What does your behavior say about your personality?
4. What characteristics do you have that you would like to keep?
5. What characteristics would you like to develop?

**Leadership Considerations:**
1. The leader should encourage the teams to discuss their answer to the game and come to a team consensus before anyone shouts out the answer.
2. The leader should praise the teams that are following directions and working as a group.

**Variations:**
1. The participants may make up a situation to give to the other team for a grand finale round.
2. The leader may alter the content area, e.g., social skills.

**Creator:** Amanda L. McGowen, Illinois State University, Normal, Illinois.

# Save Earth!

**Space Requirements:** Classroom or activity room with a table

**Equipment/Resource Requirements:** Poster board or large paper, $8\frac{1}{2}$-by-11-inch paper, several magazines, scissors, glue, writing utensils (crayons, markers, pencils, pens)

**Group Size:** Small group

**Program Goals:**
1. To increase participants' ability to identify positive benefits of life and Earth.
2. To increase participants' ability to use positive ideas.
3. To increase participants' ability to work toward one goal.

**Program Description:**
**Preparation:**
The leader will tape paper or poster board to the table and have chairs evenly spaced around the paper.

**Introduction:**
The purpose of the activity is to have the participants understand the positive characteristics of life and Earth and work together toward one main goal.

The introduction can go as follows:

An alien ship has landed on Earth. You as human beings have to save the Earth. The aliens are from the planet Zanbog. They are traveling through our galaxy and have the power to destroy Earth. They do not see any good in Earth. We as human beings have to prove our worthy existence. We need to make a sign that says good things about Earth. Now as a group we can only make one sign. So we need to work well together and fast. The alien ship is landing in (location) on (date of activity). We need to hurry or we will be disintegrated.

**Activity Description:**
This activity will show the benefits of life and Earth. The leader will read the introduction to the activity. The leader will explain to the participants that it is important that they save the Earth and that they have to do it as a group. They need to make a sign to the aliens that explains why Earth is good. The group can make the sign by drawing or cutting from magazines. The group needs to work together to create the sign. The design on the sign has to be a group consensus. They all have to decide on one design.

Once the poster is done, each participant will write a list of what is on the poster on another piece of paper. After each participant has completed his or her list, the leader will discuss why the Earth should be saved. Also, the leader will discuss the benefits of positive things in life.

**Debriefing Questions/Closure:**
1. Can someone tell the group why the planet Earth is important?
2. Why is it important for people to work together?
3. What is one positive thing about the planet Earth?
4. What would you do if Earth was threatened by aliens?
5. What are some important things on Earth worth saving?
6. How can you help Earth be a more positive place to be?

**Leadership Considerations:**
1. The group members must be able to work safely with scissors.
2. The leader may give an example of a positive thing on Earth (e.g., mountains, people, water).

3. The leader may have group members discuss their design before drawing or pasting.

**Variations:**
1. If the only goal is to identify positive things in life, each participant can have his or her own space on the sign.

2. The leader may choose to use small sheets of paper and have the participants each draw his or her own sign.

**Creator:** Courtney Stauffer, Illinois State University, Normal, Illinois.

# Can I Be a Superhero?

**Space Requirements:** Classroom or activity room with a table

**Equipment/Resource Requirements:** Crayons, markers, colored pencils, sheets of drawing paper

**Group Size:** Small group

**Program Goals:**
1. To increase participants' ability to identify personal strengths.
2. To increase participants' ability to identify their personal potential.

**Program Description:**
**Preparation:**
The leader will gather the supplies, including two sheets of paper for every participant. The leader will prepare the activity area by spreading the crayons, markers, and pencils out on the table.

**Introduction:**
The purpose of this activity is to identify personal potential and strengths. The leader will explain the purpose and procedures to the group. The following is a suggested introduction:

Can somebody give an example of a superhero? What makes him or her a superhero? Do we have the same characteristics as a superhero? Now on the paper in front of you, draw what you would look like if you were a superhero.

**Activity Description:**
The leader will pass out a piece of paper and some writing utensils to each participant and explain the activity. If the participants could be a superhero, who would they want to be? The participants need to make up their own hero and identify his or her positive qualities. What qualities will make him or her super? The participants will take time to draw the superhero. The leader may offer assistance with writing and spelling if needed.

After all the participants have finished drawing, they will take a second piece of paper and draw a picture of themselves. There they will list all the good qualities they have and draw a picture of themselves.

After they complete their second drawing, they will explain the differences and similarities between themselves and the superhero. The activity will close with the following debriefing questions. The leader should refocus on the goals of the activity.

**Debriefing Questions/Closure:**
1. What makes a superhero super?
2. What are some good qualities you have?
3. How are they different from the superhero's?
4. If you had to pick a positive quality you wanted but don't have now, what would it be?
5. What would your name be if you were a superhero?

**Leadership Considerations:**
1. The leader should draw a picture of what he or she would look like as a superhero and use it for an example.
2. If all the participants are comfortable, have them all read aloud the differences between their superhero and themselves.

**Variations:**
1. Instead of drawing themselves as a superhero, the participants can pick an existing superhero.
2. If any participants are unable to draw well, the leader may have them cut pictures from magazines and comic books.

**Creator:** Courtney Stauffer, Illinois State University, Normal, Illinois.

# Who Are You?

**Space Requirements:** Classroom or activity room

**Equipment/Resource Requirements:** Magazines, scissors, glue, construction paper, colored markers

**Group Size:** Small group

**Program Goals:**
1. To increase participants' awareness of positive self characteristics.
2. To improve participants' understanding of others' attitudes, values and interests.

**Program Description:**

**Preparation:**
The leader should complete an example to share with the group.

**Introduction:**
The leader will explain to the participants that they will be doing an activity that focuses on looking at themselves, specifically their attitudes, values, interests, and/or anything else they would like to share with the group about themselves.

**Activity Description:**
The leader will distribute one large sheet of construction paper to each participant and place scissors, glue and magazines on the table, within reach of all group members. The leader will explain to the participants that they are to go through the magazines and cut out pictures that represent their attitudes, values, interests and/or anything else that is representative of their lifestyle. Clippings can range from pictures of people engaging in sports and fun activities to just words that describe themselves. If participants are unable to find a picture they would like to include, they may draw it. The leader should allow 15–20 minutes for completion of this step.

After all the participants have found at least 10 pictures, they will paste their pictures on the construction paper to form a collage. When this step is complete, each participant will share and explain his or her collage to the group.

The leader will conclude the activity by asking the following debriefing questions.

**Debriefing Questions/Closure:**
1. Did you have any problems finding pictures that represent yourself?
2. Have you ever given thought to what your attitudes, values and interests are?
3. Explain how the various items on the collage represent you.
4. How is your collage the same or different than those of other group participants?
5. What positive things does the collage say about you?

**Leadership Consideration:**
Magazines should be age-appropriate.

**Variations:**
1. The participants can divide the construction paper into two columns. One column can represent their current values, attitudes and interests. The other column can represent future values, attitudes and interests.
2. The leader may choose a different theme for the collage, e.g., only leisure interests, meanings of friendship, or family values.

**Creator:** Lazheta Thomas, Illinois State University, Normal, Illinois.

# In With the Good;
# Keep the Bad Out

**Space Requirements:** Classroom, activity room, or gymnasium

**Equipment/Resource Requirements:** Large pieces of paper (large enough to trace bodies), writing utensils

**Group Size:** Small group

**Program Goals:**
1. To increase participants' knowledge of positive aspects of healthy living.
2. To increase participants' knowledge of negative aspects of unhealthy living.

**Program Description:**
**Preparation:**
The leader will gather supplies and tape the pieces of paper to the floor to trace the participants' bodies on.

**Introduction:**
The purpose of this activity is to increase knowledge of healthy living of the body, heart, and mind. The leader may open the activity discussion with an introduction similar to the following:

> Can someone name things that are good for our bodies? Can anyone name things that are bad for our bodies? It is important that everyone listen carefully today.

**Activity Description:**
The leader will divide the group into pairs. The partners will trace each other's bodies on the paper. After this is completed the participants should sit on their tracings. This activity goes step-by-step so the participants must follow directions well. First the participants will write everything that is good for the mind inside the head of the body (e.g., learning, listening to people). Then

the participants will write everything that is bad for the mind on the outside of the traced head. Negative things (e.g., insults, bad language) are not allowed inside the head.

Next, the participants will write everything that is good for the body on the inside of the body under the chest (e.g., exercise, good food, deep breathing). Then the participants write everything that is bad for the body on the outside of the traced body under the chest (e.g., drugs, too much fat, sugar, or salt).

Last, the participants will write everything that is good for the heart on the inside of the chest (e.g., feelings and emotions such as love, contentment, and satisfaction). Then the participants will write everything that is bad for the heart on the outside of the chest outline (e.g., hate, distrust, jealousy).

After all the parts are written, the participants will discuss their comments as a group. The following questions may be used for closure.

**Debriefing Questions/Closure:**
1. Why is it important to keep bad things out of our body?
2. Why is it important to keep good things in the body?
3. Can someone tell me a good thing for the body, mind, and heart (soul)?
4. Can someone tell me a bad thing for the body, mind, and heart (soul)?
5. What do you try to keep out of your body, mind, and heart (soul)?
6. What were the similarities in participants' answers? What were the differences in participants' answers?
7. What did you learn from this activity?

**Leadership Considerations:**
1. The leader should enforce that only appropriate things will be drawn inside and outside of the bodies.

2. The leader may prepare examples of good and bad things in advance.
3. The leader may have the tracings prepared before beginning the activity.

**Variations:**

1. The focus of the activity can be on one of the three—mind, body, heart (soul)—instead of all three.
2. The participants may draw the good and bad qualities.

**Creator:** Courtney Stauffer, Illinois State University, Normal, Illinois.

# That's My Attitude

**Space Requirements:** Classroom or activity room

**Equipment/Resource Requirements:** Accompanying form, writing utensils

**Group Size:** Small group

**Program Goals:**
1. To increase participants' ability to identify different attitudes.
2. To increase participants' understanding of their own attitudes.
3. To increase participants' understanding of appropriate times for different attitudes.

**Program Description:**
**Preparation:**
The leader will have paper and writing utensils available for every participant.

**Introduction:**
The purpose of the activity is to help the participants identify different attitudes and their most typical time and place.

The following is a suggestion for introducing the activity:

What is an attitude? What are some different types? Who thinks they have an attitude here? Everyone take your paper and let's get started.

**Activity Description:**
The leader will hand out the work sheets and writing utensils to each participant. The leader will explain that there are several "right" answers to each question. Participants must complete the work sheet individually. The leader will allow 10–15 minutes for completion.

At the end of the activity, the participants will compare their attitude sheets and discuss answers. As always, the leader should offer assistance when needed.

The leader will conclude the activity by restating the goals and discussing the following debriefing questions.

**Debriefing Questions/Closure:**
1. Name three different types of attitudes.
2. What happens if you have the wrong attitude at the wrong time?
3. Give an example of when you have had a negative attitude.
4. Give an example of when you have had a positive attitude.
5. What would happen if everyone on earth had a negative attitude?
6. What does this saying mean: Attitudes are contagious, is yours worth catching?

**Leadership Considerations:**
1. The leader should give each participant a chance to share his or her answers.
2. If some of the attitudes cross over into various situations, the leader may offer an explanation as to why.

**Variation:**
The participants may act out a variety of attitude situations.

**Creator:** Courtney Stauffer, Illinois State University, Normal, Illinois.

# That's My Attitude
## Work Sheet

1. What type of attitude would you use if your were playing a sport?

2. Write as many sports as you can think of that begin with the letter *A*.

3. What type of attitude would you use if you're playing a game that you made up?

4. Write as many things as you can that you dream or imagine.

5. What type of attitude would you use if you knew you could do something really well?

6. Write as many positive words as you can think of.

7. If you were working with a group of people, what type of attitude would you need?

8. Write as many things as you can think of that you do in groups.

9. During your quiet time, what type of attitude do you need?

10. Write down as many things that are quiet that you can do during that time.

# Show Me Fitness

**Space Requirements:** Classroom or gymnasium

**Equipment/Resource Requirements:** Playing cards with fitness words written on them

**Group Size:** Small group

**Program Goals:**
1. To increase participants' knowledge of various fitness activities.
2. To increase participants' knowledge of fitness activities that can be done alone.
3. To increase participants' ability to identify the importance of fitness in everyone's lifestyle.

**Program Description:**
**Preparation:**
The leader will prepare playing cards and prepare the activity area by clearing all tables and chairs out of the way and placing the playing cards in a basket or in a pile in the middle of the floor. Examples of fitness words include:

- aerobics,
- badminton,
- baseball,
- basketball,
- dancing,
- flag football,
- football,
- hiking,
- hockey,
- in-line skating,
- jogging,
- jumping rope,
- martial arts,
- push-ups,
- roller-skating,
- running,
- sit-ups,
- skiing,
- soccer,
- softball,
- stretching,
- swimming,
- tennis,
- volleyball,
- walking, and
- weightlifting.

**Introduction:**
The purpose of the activity is to introduce participants to fitness activities as well as to assist them in identifying how fitness fits into their lifestyles.

A suggestion for introducing the activity is as follows:

Can someone name different types of fitness or exercise? How often do you usually exercise? Is exercise important? Why? We are now going to pick a card and try to act out the exercise. The rest of the group has to guess the exercise.

**Activity Description:**
The group members will sit in a circle to listen to the directions. The leader will explain that the participants will pick out a game card and act out the activity on the card. The rest of the group has to guess the fitness activity. Participants will take turns and act out one card at a time.

When all of the cards have been acted out or when time runs out, each participant will name four fitness activities that were mentioned. The leader may ask what their favorite fitness activities are. The leader concludes the session by discussing the following debriefing questions and summarizing the goals of the activity.

**Debriefing Questions/Closure:**
1. Why is fitness important in our lives?
2. What would happen if we didn't exercise?

3. Can anyone name some fitness activities that we didn't act out?
4. Which of the fitness activities could be done alone?
5. What are the benefits of exercising daily?
6. Name one activity that you could do every day for fitness.

**Leadership Considerations:**
1. The leader should keep the activity on task. The participants may like to act out more than one fitness activity at a time.
2. The leader should assist the participants if they are unfamiliar with the fitness activity.

3. The leader should offer assistance if needed to act out a fitness activity.

**Variations:**
1. The participants can make up all the fitness activities.
2. The participants can add to the existing activities.
3. The participants could be divided into teams and compete against one another.

**Creator:** Courtney Stauffer, Illinois State University, Normal, Illinois.

# Say It, Solve It Jeopardy

**Space Requirements:** Classroom or activity room

**Equipment/Resource Requirements:** Playing cards, masking tape

**Group Size:** Small group

**Program Goals:**
1. To increase participants' ability to problem solve.
2. To increase participants' ability to be assertive in a positive way.
3. To increase participants' ability to work in teams.

**Program Description:**
**Preparation:**
The leader will prepare game cards (see accompanying list for suggestions) and tape them to the wall like a game show.

**Introduction:**
The purpose of this activity is to increase participants' problem-solving and positive assertiveness skills.

A suggested introduction for the activity is as follows:

Who has ever seen the show "Jeopardy"? We are going to play a game of Jeopardy that works on problem solving and assertiveness. Can anyone tell me what assertiveness means?

**Activity Description:**
The participants will sit facing the game wall. The participants will be playing as individuals, not as teams. The leader will start the game by having a participant pick a category with point numbers. The leader will be scorekeeper.

Each participant will want to try to score a total of 600 points. The leader should restate the purpose of the game. If a participant does not answer the question appropriately the card goes back on the board. Each participant answers one question each turn.

Play continues until all the questions have been answered.

The leader will refocus on the activity goals of problem solving and assertiveness and use the following debriefing questions for closure.

**Debriefing Questions/Closure:**
1. Why is it hard to make a decision in tough situations?
2. Who considers themselves assertive already?
3. What are good ways to be assertive?
4. How could being assertive help in everyday life?
5. What is the difference between assertive and aggressive?
6. What are the benefits of being assertive?
7. What are the benefits of being able to solve your own problems?

**Leadership Considerations:**
1. The leader should be prepared to help explain what assertiveness is.
2. The leader should adjust situations to participants' understanding level.
3. The leader should make sure everyone takes at least one turn.

**Variations:**
1. The participants may make up their own situations.
2. The participants may role-play situations.
3. Additional categories can be created to fit the needs of the participants.

**Creator:** Courtney Stauffer, Illinois State University, Normal, Illinois.

# Say It, Solve It Jeopardy

*Problem Solving:*

200—What would you do if your friend was making fun of a girl?

300—What would you do if you and your friend started to argue?

400—What would you do if your friends wanted to play hooky from school?

500—What would you do if you smelled smoke in your house in the middle of the night?


*Assertiveness:*

200—How would you tell your teacher that you didn't understand what she said?

300—How would you tell your friend that she was making a big mistake?

400—How would you talk to someone who just took your book?

500—What would you say to someone who started accusing you of something you didn't do?


*Sports* (Bonus; participants can only answer one sports question):

200—Name three sports that use rackets.

200—Name three sports that are played in the water.

200—Name three sports that have a net.

200—Name two sports that use mats.

# What Are My Personal Qualities?

**Space Requirements:** Classroom or activity room

**Equipment/Resource Requirements:** Writing utensils, five pieces of string or paper brads per participant, one package of cutout shapes per participant (Package includes one head, one torso, two arms and two legs. The cutout shapes should be hole punched at the appropriate end so that they can be attached to form a person [see accompanying form].)

**Group Size:** Small group

**Program Goals:**
1. To increase participants' knowledge of positive personal characteristics.
2. To increase participants' ability to follow directions and stay on task.

**Program Description:**
**Preparation:**
The leader will gather all materials and prepare a list of 15–20 positive personal characteristics or qualities that people hold.

**Introduction:**
The leader will begin the activity by initiating a discussion on what positive personal characteristics are. The leader may ask for and provide some examples of positive characteristics or qualities that people hold. In case the participants are unable to think of many examples, the leader should already have a list of 15–20 positive personal characteristics and qualities prepared to share with the group.

Next, the leader will explain to the participants that they will be doing an activity that involves disclosing what their positive personal characteristics and qualities are. This will be done by constructing a "paper person." This person should represent the participant.

**Activity Description:**
Each participant will receive one package of cut-out shapes and a writing utensil. The leader will explain to the group members that they should choose one or two words to write on each of their cutout shapes. The words should represent positive personal characteristics or qualities that they have. The leader will explain that these words have to be qualities that they currently have and exercise. They should not be qualities the participants would like to have or begin practicing. The leader will inform the group members that later in the activity they will have to give examples of how they exercise these particular qualities. All words must be positive.

After participants have finished writing their positive qualities on their cutout shapes, the leader will distribute five pieces of string or paper brads to each participant. At this time, the participants will put "themselves" together. To do this, each will attach the head to the torso, arms to torso, and legs to torso.

After all have put "themselves" together, each participant will share his or her positive characteristics or qualities with the group. While doing this, the participants also should give an explanation or example of what actions they do to show others that they possess those qualities. The leader should encourage the other group members to ask questions that relate to the personal qualities.

The leader will close by refocusing on the activity goals and the following debriefing questions.

**Debriefing Questions/Closure:**
1. Was it easy or difficult for you to think of your positive qualities?
2. What have you learned about yourself from this activity? What have you learned about others?

3. If you could do this activity again, say in three months, what particular positive characteristics or qualities would you like to add?
4. Why is it important to recognize positive qualities in yourself and others?
5. Name one personal quality that you're really proud of.

**Leadership Consideration:**
The leader should make sure all qualities discussed are positive in nature.

**Variations:**
1. The participants may make two "paper persons"—one of current characteristics they possess and another of future characteristics or qualities they would like to possess.
2. The leader may have a variety of additional craft and art supplies available for participants to decorate "themselves," e.g., googly eyes, yarn for hair, fabric scraps for clothes.
3. Instead of making a "paper person" of themselves, the participants may make a person to represent their role model.

**Creator:** Lazheta Thomas, Illinois State University, Normal, Illinois.

# What Are My Personal Qualities?

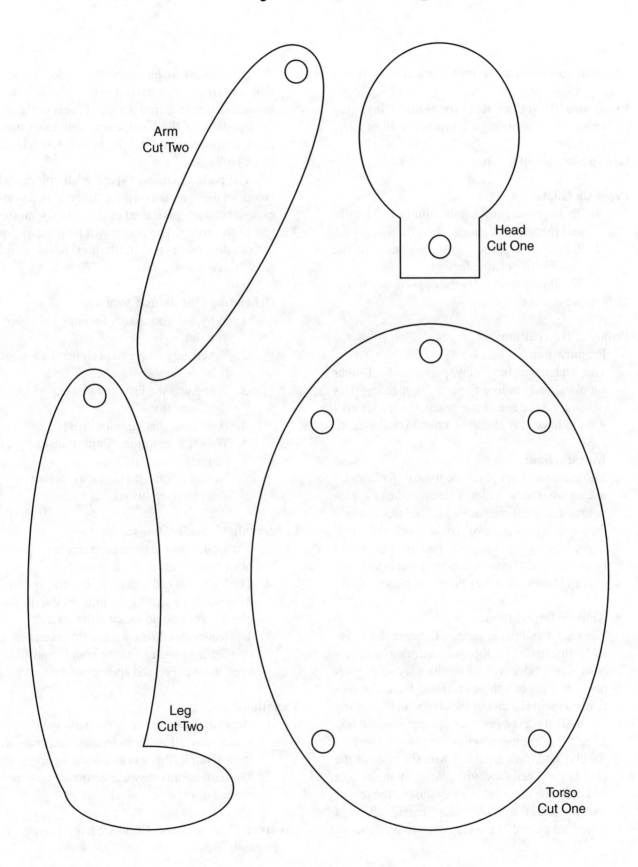

Arm
Cut Two

Head
Cut One

Leg
Cut Two

Torso
Cut One

# Feelings Fingers

**Space Requirements:** Art room with clay oven

**Equipment/Resource Requirements:** Clay, clay knives, acrylic paint, paintbrushes, rolling pins

**Group Size:** Small group

**Program Goals:**
1. To improve participants' ability to identify and recognize feelings.
2. To improve participants' awareness of the benefits of positive feelings.
3. To allow participants the opportunity to express creativity.

**Program Description:**
**Preparation:**
The leader will have clay, paints and all other supplies ready before the activity meeting. Depending on the age of the group, the leader may want to have clay already sectioned or flattened.

**Introduction:**
The leader will introduce the topic of feelings by asking what some feelings are and when the participants may experience them. The leader should distinguish between positive and negative feelings and why they are such. Participants should be encouraged to give examples of individual feelings and times when they have experienced them.

**Activity Description:**
The leader and participants will begin the activity by discussing the topic of feelings as a group. Next, the leader will distribute clay to participants and explain the directions. First, the participants will flatten out the clay with the rolling pin until the clay is about one-half-inch thick. Then the participants will each place a hand on the clay and trace around it with the edge of the clay knife. Then they will take away their hand and continue to cut all the way though the rest of the clay until they have a clay "hand." The clay hands are placed in the clay oven to harden.

Once hands are hardened and cooled the participants will paint each finger the color of a different emotion (e.g., red is anger, blue is sadness). On the palm of the hand, each participant may paint any situation when he or she felt one of these feelings.

The participants will share what colors and emotions they painted on their "fingers" and what experiences are portrayed in the palms with the rest of the group. The leader will help the group discuss differences and similarities, positive and negative emotions.

**Debriefing Questions/Closure:**
1. Why did you assign feelings the colors you did?
2. When have you experienced each of these feelings?
3. When was the last time you experienced these emotions?
4. How does that emotion feel?
5. Why are emotions important to us as people?
6. How can you tell a positive emotion from a negative emotion?

**Leadership Considerations:**
1. The leader should have an example prepared prior to the start of the activity.
2. The leader should supervise the activity carefully so there will be no injuries due to the clay knives and no major paint spills.
3. The leader should emphasize that even negative feelings such as anger aren't "bad," but need to be expressed appropriately.

**Variations:**
1. Depending on the age of the participants, the leader may allow them to make clay dough from scratch (this works similar to clay).
2. The participants may use construction paper instead of clay.

**Creator:** Kristen Boys, Illinois State University, Normal, Illinois.

# Animated Names

**Space Requirements:** Classroom or activity room

**Equipment/Resource Requirements:** Colored construction paper, markers, pencils, colored pencils, scissors, glue, white drawing paper

**Group Size:** Small group

**Program Goals:**
1. To increase participants' awareness of personal traits.
2. To increase participants' ability to recognize similarities and/or differences among peers.
3. To increase participants' ability to follow sequenced directions.

**Program Description:**
**Preparation:**
All materials should be placed in the center of the tables prior to the start of the activity. The leader should prepare an example of both a name and drawings prior to the start of the activity.

**Introduction:**
The leader will explain to the group that this activity involves creativity and the ability to identify personal traits. The leader will explain that the traits seen in different animals will be used as examples and inspirations to aid the participants in identifying their own personal traits.

**Activity Description:**
Using their first name, the participants will choose one animal for each letter in their first name. The animals chosen should represent or have a similar character trait as the participant, for example:

T—Tiger
E—Eagle
R—Rabbit
R—Raccoon
I—Iguana

Once the animals have been chosen, the participants are to draw each animal. Participants should be encouraged to use all materials provided—animals can be cut out and glued to another page; pictures can be freestanding; or pictures can be made into a poster or an advertisement.

Once all names have been "animated," the participants will share what animals they chose and the reasons they chose those particular animals.

The leader will use the following debriefing questions to refocus on the goals of the activity.

**Debriefing Questions/Closure:**
1. What are the letters in your name?
2. What animal did you choose for each letter?
3. How do the animals you chose represent something about you?
4. What was difficult about identifying animals that have traits similar to yours? What was easy?
5. Which traits represented are positive?
6. How are your traits similar to or different from others in the group?
7. What did you learn by doing this activity?

**Leadership Considerations:**
1. The leader should have a list of animals prepared for each letter of the alphabet.
2. If a participant's first name is short (less than three letters), the participant should use his or her last name.

3. Participants may use stencils, if available.
4. The leader may prepare an example prior to the start of the activity.

**Variations:**

1. The participants may use languages and cultures to spell and animate names, for example:

   R—Romanian
   I—Incan
   C—Chinese
   H—Hindi

2. The leader may allow the participants to use only certain animals from specific locations such as the zoo, the ocean, or the jungle to animate their names.
3. The participants may make the letters or drawings three-dimensional.
4. The participants may use traits they would like to develop instead of ones they have now.

**Creator:** Theresa M. Connolly, CTRS, Illinois State University, Normal, Illinois.

# Junk Collage

**Space Requirements:** Classroom or activity room

**Equipment/Resource Requirements:** Copy of poem "Sarah Cynthia Sylvia Stout Would Not Take the Garbage Out" by Shel Silverstein (from *Where the Sidewalk Ends: The Poems and Drawings of Shel Silverstein* published in 1974 by Harper-Collins), bags to collect garbage, collected pieces of garbage, a large sheet of paper, glue, markers

**Group Size:** Small group

**Program Goals:**
1. To improve participants' awareness of the need for cleanliness.
2. To improve participants' ability to identify appropriate ways to increase cleanliness within their daily living.

**Program Description:**
**Preparation:**
The leader will have all supplies available ahead of time and obtain a copy of the poem "Sarah Cynthia Sylvia Stout Would Not Take the Garbage Out."

**Introduction:**
The purpose of this activity is to provide participants with the opportunity to increase their knowledge of cleanliness habits and the importance of cleanliness, while identifying appropriate ways to increase cleanliness within their daily living habits.

**Activity Description:**
The leader should state goals and purpose of the activity, then read the poem, "Sarah Cynthia Sylvia Stout Would Not Take the Garbage Out" by Shel Silverstein. The leader should involve participants in a discussion about the poem and important cleanliness habits.

The leader should state instructions for the activity. Participants will search the area for pieces of garbage that they can include on the mural and place it in their bag. The leader should give some examples of acceptable and nonacceptable pieces of garbage to collect.

Participants will work together to make a large collection of the items collected. Then, they will glue the items on the large paper as a mural. The leader should encourage the participants to think of a title for the mural.

The leader will end the activity with a discussion about the importance of cleanliness.

**Debriefing Questions/Closure:**
1. What did you learn about cleanliness?
2. What actions can you take to be neater?
3. Why is cleanliness important?
4. What would happen if we never took the garbage out?
5. What would happen if we never cleaned our rooms?

**Leadership Considerations:**
1. The leader should tell the participants that they are not to pick up any sharp or dangerous objects.
2. The leader should tell the participants that they are only to use objects that fit in their bag.
3. The leader should tell the participants that they are not to pull up any plants or to include any animals in their bag.
4. The leader should encourage participants to search for the oddest piece of garbage. Also, the leader may have participants see who can collect the most garbage.
5. The leader should encourage participants to share materials and work together.

**Variations:**

1. The participants could create a garbage sculpture.
2. The leader may choose to have a Garbage Treasure Hunt. The leader should prepare a list of garbage items ahead of time and have the participants search for garbage. When they have collected all their garbage, they will sit in a circle. The leader will stand in the center of the circle. The leader will call out an item and the first person to show the item will receive a point. The person with the most points will receive a prize.

**Creator:** Renee Raczkowski, Illinois State University, Normal, Illinois.

# Feelings Mobile

**Space Requirements:** Classroom or activity room

**Equipment/Resource Requirements:** List of feelings, markers, construction paper, dowel rods or straws, string, hole puncher

**Group Size:** Small group

**Program Goals:**
1. To improve participants' ability to identify different feelings within their life.
2. To improve participants' ability to express verbally their feelings.
3. To improve participants' knowledge of ways to express appropriately their feelings.

**Program Description:**
**Preparation:**
The leader should have face shapes precut and hole punched. Situations should be prepared ahead of time. The leader also should have mobile tops made and string cut.

**Introduction:**
The purpose of this activity is to provide participants with the opportunity to develop knowledge of feelings, and identify and verbally express feelings appropriately within their life.

**Activity Description:**
The leader begins by stating the goals and purpose of the activity. The leader will hold a discussion on what feelings are, and what feelings one has in one's life. Examples of feelings include:

- angry,
- anxious,
- bored,
- content,
- excited,
- frustrated,
- guilty

- happy,
- sad,
- satisfied, and
- upset.

Each participant will receive four to eight precut face shapes. The participants will decorate and color the faces to express different feelings. Participants will be given a situation, and they must hold up the face that expresses how the situation makes them feel. Participants may discuss reasons for choosing the face they did.

Next, the participants will draw a picture on the back of each face of when they experience this feeling the most. When completed, the participants will create a mobile of their completed faces to hang in their rooms.

The leader will hold a discussion about what the participants learned about feelings and how they can appropriately express these feelings. The leader will restate the goals and purpose of the activity. The leader may use the following debriefing questions to reemphasize goals of the activity.

**Debriefing Questions/Closure:**
1. What feeling do you experience most often?
2. What makes you feel this way?
3. What makes you feel happy? Sad? Angry? Scared?
4. How can you appropriately express your feelings?
5. When should you express feelings and when should you control feelings?

**Leadership Considerations:**
1. The leader should encourage participants to think about how the situation would really make them feel.
2. The leader should emphasize that there is no right or wrong answer.

3. The leader should encourage participants to be creative in decorating their faces to look how they feel by using colors that may relate to the feeling.
4. The leader should encourage participants to be considerate of others' feelings.

**Variations:**
1. Participants can create a mobile of favorite leisure activities.
2. A mobile of leisure resources can be created.

**Creator:** Renee Raczkowski, Illinois State University, Normal, Illinois.

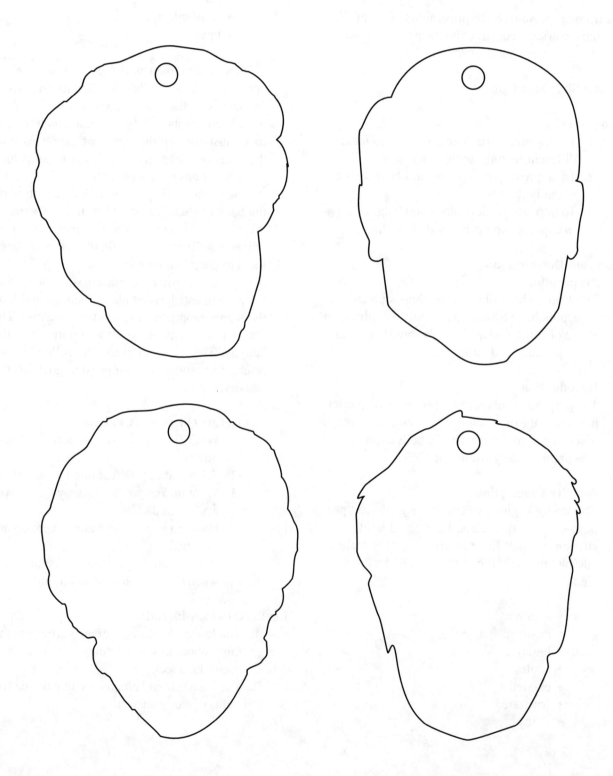

# Search for Your Emotions

**Space Requirements:** Classroom or activity room with desks or tables

**Equipment/Resource Requirements:** Work sheet prepared by leader, writing utensils

**Group Size:** Any

**Program Goals:**
1. To increase participants' awareness of feelings and emotions.
2. To introduce feelings and emotions that participants may be unfamiliar with.
3. To increase participants' concentration levels.

**Program Description:**
**Preparation:**
The leader should create a word search, using words understood by participants (see the accompanying list). The leader should make one copy for each participant. Emotions for the word search could include:

- anger,
- boredom,
- excitement,
- fear,
- guilt,
- happiness,
- hate,
- love,
- resentment,
- sadness, and
- satisfaction.

**Introduction:**
The leader will explain the importance of expressing emotions. The leader will explain that when a person is in touch with his or her feelings, it makes it easier to talk about tough, sad, and happy times in his or her life. It also makes it much easier to talk to someone else who is experiencing different emotions or feelings.

**Activity Description:**
The leader will distribute the word search and discuss each word so that participants are clear on the meaning. The leader will give the participants a time limit for completion of the word search. The group will discuss the following closure questions.

**Debriefing Questions/Closure:**
1. What are some other emotions or feelings that you could add to the word search?
2. Have you experienced any of these feelings? Which ones? Which emotions have you never felt?
3. Can you think of an event that would make you experience one of these emotions?
4. Do you think any of these emotions can be felt at the same time? How?
5. Do you see any of these emotions as uncool or inappropriate? Which ones?

**Leadership Considerations:**
1. The leader should have discussion ideas ready ahead of time covering as many emotions as possible.
2. The leader should allow enough time for discussion after the word searches are completed.
3. The leader should use participant examples of emotions they experience to initiate conversation about personal feelings.

**Variations:**
1. The leader may choose not to provide a list of the words to be found. Instead, the leader may put them on cards and have each participant pick a card and make a facial expression to match the emotion. When the rest of the participants guess it, they may add it to their word search list.

2. Along with the word search, the leader may pass out a number of cartoon faces with facial expressions depicting emotions. The participants will figure out the emotions and add them to their list of words to find.

3. The participants may make their own word search using emotions or feelings that they have personally experienced.

**Creator:** Kristen Boys, Illinois State University, Normal, Illinois.

# Who Would You Be?

**Space Requirements:** Classroom or activity room

**Equipment/Resource Requirements:** Crayons or markers, accompanying form

**Group Size:** Small group

**Program Goals:**
1. To increase participants' ability to identify positive role models.
2. To increase participants' ability to identify positive personal characteristics of role models.

**Program Description:**
**Preparation:**
The leader should gather supplies and make one copy of the accompanying form per participant.

**Introduction:**
This activity is designed to encourage participants to identify positive personal characteristics and associate those with characteristics of their role models.

**Activity Description:**
The leader will begin the activity by discussing what role models are and why they are a good thing to have. Next, the leader will distribute one work sheet to each participant. Once everyone receives a work sheet, the leader will instruct the participants to read through each of the categories on the work sheet and identify a role model for each category. The role model should represent someone whom they admire and wish to be like. The leader should discourage the participants from identifying villains or "bad guys."

After identifying a role model for each category, each participant will write down the name of that role model in the respective category.

Next, the participants will draw a picture of that role model. Below each picture, they will write two or more positive qualities that this role model has. The characteristics should represent what has attracted the participants to them, and what made them want to be like the role models.

Once everyone has completed the activity, each participant will tell the group who it is he or she looks up to and why he or she would like to be more like this person.

**Debriefing Questions/Closure:**
1. What positive qualities do your role models have?
2. What positive qualities do you share with your role model in each category?
3. What positive qualities do you need to develop to be a role model?
4. How did you select your role models?

**Leadership Considerations:**
1. The leader should not allow participants to choose villains or "bad guys" as their role models.
2. The leader should be prepared to give examples of positive qualities that a person might have.

**Variations:**
1. The participants may do the activity and draw a character that they are most like, and one that they wish to be most like. The participants will compare and contrast the two.
2. The leader may alter the content of the categories to include people they interact with on a daily, weekly, or monthly basis.

**Creator:** Jessica Kamm, Illinois State University, Normal, Illinois.

# Who Would You Be?

Cartoon Character                                    Superhero



Musician                                             Football Player



Movie Star                                           Basketball Player



Baseball Player                                      Anyone in the World

# Cooperation, Communication, and Listening Skills

# Snake Pit

**Space Requirements:** Large activity room or gymnasium

**Equipment/Resource Requirements:** Jump ropes, cones, obstacles of any kind, blindfold

**Group Size:** Small group

**Program Goals:**
1. To increase participants' ability to work with a partner.
2. To develop participants' sense of trust in a partner.

**Program Description:**
**Preparation:**
The leader will prepare the room by setting up one boundary on each side of the room (like a goal line) and scattering obstacles (e.g., cones, jump ropes, balls) around the middle area. This serves as the Snake Pit. To make it challenging for each person, the leader may choose to rearrange the obstacles each time a new participant goes through.

**Introduction:**
The leader will introduce participants to trust and teamwork activities in an active environment. The leader and the group will discuss the importance of teamwork and trust. They also will discuss the importance of good communication and listening skills. The leader should be prepared to go through a trial run as an example.

**Activity Description:**
The activity leader can either assign partners or allow participants to select partners. One partner will be blindfolded for his or her turn.

The pair leader (nonblindfolded partner) will verbally direct his or her partner through the Snake Pit. The pair leader may not touch the blindfolded partner; all communication must be verbal. Other participants may cheer on the pair, therefore forcing the blindfolded partner to have to listen very carefully to the pair leader.

If any of the "snakes" are touched by either of the participants, the pair must return to the start and try again to get through the pit. Once the first pair have gone through, two more participants may begin.

The leader will close the activity by having participants sit in a circle, and discuss the following questions.

**Debriefing Questions/Closure:**
1. What was it like to rely on your partner to get you through the Snake Pit?
2. How easy or difficult was it to trust your partner?
3. What helps build trust? What prevents or decreases trust?
4. How did you feel as a leader or as a follower?
5. Do you prefer being a leader or a follower? Why?
6. Why are good listening skills important for this activity?
7. What did you learn from this activity?
8. How will you use what you've learned?

**Leadership Considerations:**
1. The activity leader should have the Snake Pit set up prior to activity time.
2. The activity leader should give suggestions on how to be a good leader and/or follower, through the Snake Pit.

**Variations:**
1. The participants may attempt the Snake Pit alone with no verbal help from a partner.
2. The leader may set a time limit for the Snake Pit. As the participants get better at communicating and trusting, he or she will shorten the limit.

**Creator:** Kristen Boys, Illinois State University, Normal, Illinois.

# Team Puzzling

**Space Requirements:** Classroom or activity room with large tables

**Equipment/Resource Requirements:** One 500-piece jigsaw puzzle per four participants, large surface area to work puzzle on (puzzle may be smaller than 500 pieces, depending on participants, but must remain very challenging)

**Group Size:** Minimum of 8 participants

**Program Goals:**
1. To increase participants' ability to work as a team member.
2. To increase participants' knowledge of a leisure activity (puzzles).

**Program Description:**

**Preparation:**
The leader should make sure that puzzles include all pieces (there's nothing more frustrating than finishing and realizing there's one piece missing!). Also, the leader should ensure that if puzzles are left overnight they will not be disturbed.

**Introduction:**
The leader will present to the group the concept that putting together jigsaw puzzles is a great way to spend free time instead of less constructive alternatives. Putting together puzzles also is a great way to spend a rainy Saturday with family or friends. The leader will introduce this activity as a friendly competition between two teams. Prizes should not be awarded. The goal is to finish the puzzle in the shortest amount of time possible.

**Activity Description:**
The leader will assign teams and distribute one jigsaw puzzle to each team. The leader should designate certain "puzzle times," for example, lunch breaks and recess. The leader should set a few guidelines, for example no more than four people at a puzzle table at one time (it can get extremely crowded), no touching other group members, and no touching the other group's puzzle.

Once a puzzle has been completed, the participants may disassemble and switch puzzles with another group. When the time allotted for the activity is nearly done, the teams will come together as a group and discuss how the groups felt they did on the teamwork aspect. They may discuss the following questions.

**Debriefing Questions/Closure:**
1. Who emerged as the leader of your group? Why?
2. What feelings did doing the jigsaw puzzle evoke: anger, frustration, sense of accomplishment?
3. How did you and your group deal with those feelings?
4. How did each of you contribute to your group?
5. What did you learn about teamwork from this activity?
6. How will you use this information in the future?

**Leadership Consideration:**
The leader should downplay the competition between teams. The leader should encourage quiet work and stress the leisure aspect of doing a jigsaw puzzle.

**Variations:**
1. The leader may allow the participants to research and make their own puzzles out of clay, cardboard or tagboard. Then they can exchange puzzles with others and compare their difficulty.
2. The leader may introduce other quiet leisure games that can be done alone or with others.

**Creator:** Kristen Boys, Illinois State University, Normal, Illinois.

# Be Clear!

**Space Requirements:** Classroom or activity room

**Equipment/Resource Requirements:** Cards with geometric shapes or figures on them, writing utensils, paper

**Group Size:** Small group

**Program Goals:**
1. To improve participants' descriptive communication skills.
2. To provide an opportunity for participants to give and follow instructions.
3. To enhance participants' listening skills.

**Program Description:**
**Preparation:**
The leader should create or locate cards with geometric shapes printed on them prior to the start of the activity.

**Introduction:**
As soon as participants enter the room, the leader will give them a set of directions that are intentionally indecisive and unclear; for example, too many directions at once, directions given too fast, and asking them to do something they do not know how to do.

When participants look confused, the leader will ask them what was difficult about following the directions. Following this, the leader will explain the importance of expressing oneself so that others can understand the message. The leader will explain that listening carefully to each person's description of the shape will be very important to the outcome of the drawings. The leader will ask the participants to give better examples of the directions he or she gave at the start of the session.

**Activity Description:**
Participant number one will pick a card with a geometric shape on it from the leader. The individual with the card will give the other partici-

pants only verbal directions on how to draw the shape, without naming the shape. Participants are not allowed to ask questions and must work alone.

When everyone is done, the individual with the card will disclose the original drawing to the others to compare their drawing to the actual shape. Each person should have at least one chance to describe a shape. The leader should allow time for discussion of closure questions after each participant has been given the opportunity to instruct.

**Debriefing Questions/Closure:**
1. How easy or difficult was it to understand other people's directions?
2. How important were good listening skills?
3. What helped make the directions clear when you had to draw the object?
4. What are your suggestions for clear communication?
5. Discuss a situation in everyday life where clear communication is important.
6. How can you use what you learned today in improving your communication?

**Leadership Considerations:**
1. The leader should use the first set of directions (see Introduction) as an example of what not to do.
2. The leader should provide ample time for discussion of each drawing.

**Variations:**
1. After completing this activity, the participants will split into two groups and each person will draw a figure. They will give the picture to someone else in the same group who will write the directions. Then, they will give only the directions to a member of the opposite group who will make a drawing based on the directions. The participants will compare the results with the original drawing.

2. The leader may give each group instructions for a figure. He or she will set a time limit and see how the group works together in order to form the final figure.

3. For an extra challenge, the leader may add colors to the figures or time limits on the groups or individuals.

**Creator:** Kristen Boys, Illinois State University, Normal, Illinois.

# Trust Your Partner

**Space Requirements:** Gymnasium or area where there is room to move safely and freely

**Equipment/Resource Requirements:** Blindfolds and various sporting and recreational equipment that can be used as obstacles to maneuver around

**Group Size:** Small group

**Program Goals:**
1. To increase participants' ability to give and receive accurate directions in a positive manner.
2. To increase participants' ability to work cooperatively with peers.
3. To increase participants' listening skills.

**Program Description:**
**Preparation:**
The playing area should be set up ahead of time. Enough obstacles should be provided so that the course is challenging to the group. Questions should be made up ahead of time. (This activity is similar to Snake Pit, but requires more discussion between participants.)

**Introduction:**
The leader will introduce the activity to the participants by explaining that they will be playing two roles: leader and team player. For each of these roles it will be necessary for them to exercise good listening skills and good communication skills. The leader will initiate a discussion on the importance of giving accurate directions and the importance of exercising good listening skills. The leader may ask for, or provide examples of, times and events when it is important to use these skills.

The leader should tie the discussion into the topic of trust. The leader may ask each participant to define the term *trust*. Next, the leader may have each person explain how he or she has learned to trust another individual and why trust is important.

**Activity Description:**
The leader will pair participants and give each pair a blindfold. Next, the leader will explain the directions of the activity. Each person will take a turn being blindfolded. The person who is not blindfolded will be leading the other person through the danger field (obstacle course). The activity leader should decide ahead of time what type of leadership will be allowed, i.e., only verbal directions, or guidance by only holding on to partner's arm. Only one pair will go at a time.

Before the partner in the leadership role directs his or her partner through the danger field, the activity leader will ask the person wearing the blindfold a question or give the person a simple directive. This question must be answered correctly before the pair can proceed through the danger field. The partner is not allowed to offer any assistance in answering the question.

Example questions and directives (related to social skills) are:

1. Give your partner a compliment.
2. What do you say to someone who opens a door for you?
3. How would you initiate conversation with a new kid at school?

Throughout the danger field, the pair will be required to stop at certain areas so that the activity leader can ask the blindfolded partner additional questions. The activity leader should set up three to five question stations. Again, the blindfolded partner must answer these questions correctly before continuing.

While traveling through the danger zone, the pair cannot touch any of the obstacles. If they do, they must go to the end of the line and try again after all other pairs have taken their turn.

Once the pair reaches the safe zone (zone to be designated by the activity leader), they are considered to be out of harm's way.

This process should continue until each participant has had an opportunity to play both leader and team player. The leader will conclude the activity by discussing the following questions.

**Debriefing Questions/Closure:**
1. How did it feel to lead? How did it feel to be led?
2. What role did accurate communication play?
3. How important were good listening skills?
4. What was easy or difficult about the activity?
5. What did you learn from this activity?
6. How will you use what you have learned?

**Leadership Considerations:**
1. The leader should explain the directions of the activity before entering the activity area. The partner to be blindfolded will enter with the blindfold in place.
2. It may be necessary to have another supervisor in the activity room to watch participants who are waiting in line. If this is not possible, the leader may have the participants do a related activity while waiting in line.

**Variation:**
The leader may make the questions relate to a specific theme, i.e., leisure resources or leisure barriers.

**Creator:** Connie Campbell, Illinois State University, Normal, Illinois.

# Roadblocks to Communication

**Space Requirements:** Classroom or activity room

**Equipment/Resource Requirements:** Drawing paper, pencils, markers, crayons

**Group Size:** Small group

**Program Goals:**
1. To increase participants' awareness of typical blocks that interfere with successful communication.
2. To increase participants' ability to discuss communication skills with peers.
3. To improve participants' ability to follow directions.

**Program Description:**
**Preparation:**
The leader should have a completed example of the activity for demonstration purposes.

**Introduction:**
The two main purposes of this activity are (1) to increase participants' ability to identify "roadblocks" which may have a negative effect on communication, and (2) to increase participants' ability to discuss appropriate communication skills with peers.

**Activity Description:**
The leader will distribute materials (paper and writing utensil) to each participant. The participants will write a list of five "roadblocks" that have affected the success of their communication with others. This should be written in the upper left-hand corner of the page.

Next, the participants will draw a picture of a road with five detours. Each of the detours should lead back to the main road, traveling down the middle of their page. Once the roads have been designed, the participants will write *sender* at the bottom of the road, and *receiver* at the top of the road.

Now the task of each person is to draw his or her five roadblocks at the five detours on the page. The participants should draw an example of when and how each roadblock occurred and a picture that represents each roadblock. Each person should have five drawings on his or her page. *Note:* The leader should remind participants to draw small enough so all pictures can fit on the page.

The leader may conclude the activity by holding a discussion using the following questions.

**Debriefing Questions/Closure:**
1. What are the five roadblocks you listed?
2. Name times in your life when these roadblocks have occurred.
3. How could these roadblocks have been avoided?
4. Name some times in your life when you have felt misunderstood. What were the roadblocks in the communication that caused the misunderstanding?
5. What are some ways to avoid roadblocks in the future?
6. How can you apply this activity to your future communications?

**Leadership Considerations:**
1. The leader should have a prepared example of how the roadblocks and detours might look.
2. The leader should have several prepared examples of what roadblocks to communication are to aid participants.
3. If participants are unsure or uncomfortable with their drawing skills, the leader may allow them to write words or use symbols of roadblocks.

**Variations:**
1. The participants may draw two pictures: roadblocks set out by sender, roadblocks set out by receiver.

2. The leader may have the group work on a large collage of roadblocks.

3. The leader may change the theme to roadblocks to making friends, roadblocks to having successful relationships, or other roadblocks.

**Creator:** Theresa M. Connolly, CTRS, Illinois State University, Normal, Illinois.

# Blindfolded Shape Descriptions

**Space Requirements:** Classroom or activity room

**Equipment/Resource Requirements:** Several odd-shaped items, one blindfold, box

**Group Size:** Small group

**Program Goals:**
1. To improve participants' listening skills.
2. To increase participants' use of effective communication skills.
3. To increase participants' ability to problem solve.

**Program Description:**
**Preparation:**
The leader needs to gather several unusual and odd-shaped items. These need to be hidden in a box away from the participants' view.

**Introduction:**
The purpose of this activity is to increase the participants' awareness of the importance of listening and to improve the participants' ability to verbally communicate.

**Activity Description:**
The participants will sit in a circle. The leader will inform the group that each participant will take a turn being blindfolded. When the first chosen participant is blindfolded, an object will be verbally described to the blindfolded individual by the rest of the group. The group members will take turns giving one-word descriptions of the object to the blindfolded individual. The blindfolded participant may guess at any time what the object is, and if the guess is incorrect, the group will continue to give clues until the correct answer is given.

Once the object is correctly named, the blindfold will be passed to another group member and the process will be repeated with a new object so

that everyone has at least one turn at being blindfolded.

The leader will close the activity with a discussion about communication, listening, and problem-solving skills.

**Debriefing Questions/Closure:**
1. How did it feel to be blindfolded?
2. How did it feel to be responsible for describing the object?
3. Was it difficult to think of one-word descriptions without naming the object?
4. Name a time when you communicated to others using only one word or not describing the whole picture.
5. Why are listening skills important?
6. Why are effective communication skills important?
7. How does our communication affect others' perceptions of what we say?
8. How can you improve communication skills so the information you share with others will not be misunderstood?
9. What did you learn from this activity?
10. How will you use what you have learned?

**Leadership Considerations:**
1. The leader should ensure that the clues are one-word descriptions and that the name of the object is not given away.
2. The blindfolded participant may not touch the object to aid in guessing.
3. The leader should keep all unused objects hidden at all times. The only object that may be seen is the one being described.
4. The leader should allow participants to close their eyes if they are not comfortable wearing a blindfold.

**Variations:**
1. The participants may describe a location rather than an object.

2. The participants may describe a photograph rather than an object.
3. The participants may observe what others in the group are wearing and describe objects being worn by another individual. The blindfolded individual must guess who is wearing the object being described.

**Creator:** Theresa M. Connolly, CTRS, Illinois State University, Normal, Illinois.

# Group Formation

**Space Requirements:** Classroom or activity room (need ample space for participants to move around freely)

**Equipment/Resource Requirements:** Blindfolds (one per participant), long ropes or strings (ends tied together)

**Group Size:** Small group

**Program Goals:**
1. To increase participants' listening skills.
2. To improve participants' ability to follow directions given by a peer.
3. To increase participants' ability to give clear and precise directions to others.

**Program Description:**
**Preparation:**
The leader needs to prepare ropes and have ideas for how they will be shaped.

**Introduction:**
The purpose of this activity is to increase participants' ability to work cooperatively with peers while improving the ability to provide as well as follow verbal directions.

**Activity Description:**
The activity leader will explain to the participants that this activity will involve wearing blindfolds and following directions given by peers. The activity leader will divide the group into pairs. One individual in each pair will be chosen as the leader and the other will be blindfolded. The activity leader may assist the blindfolded individual in grabbing and holding the rope in his or her hands.

The activity leader will draw a shape on a board or whisper the shape into the pair leader's (nonblindfolded partner's) ear. It is the responsibility of the pair leader to verbally instruct the blindfolded partner to arrange the rope or string into specific positions so that once all are in place the rope will be in the correct shape.

The activity leader will inform the blindfolded individual that he or she is not allowed to speak and should listen carefully to the pair leader's directions. The activity leader will remind the pair leader that he or she must give only verbal directions and may not touch the blindfolded individual's rope or string. The activity leader should allow no more than five minutes for the direction-giving period. Once all the ropes are in position or time is up, the blindfolded partners may remove the blindfold and view the shape of their strings. The pairs should switch leader and blindfolded partner positions so that all individuals are able to be the leader at least once.

The activity leader will end the activity with a discussion about the importance of clear communication. The activity leader will use the following questions for debriefing.

**Debriefing Questions/Closure:**
1. How did it feel to be the leader? Did your partner follow your instructions? Were directions easy or difficult to give?
2. How did it feel being the blindfolded individual? Were the instructions easy or difficult to follow?
3. How did it feel to rely on another person for directions? Did you trust the leader?
4. What type of directions needed to be given in order for the activity to be successful?
5. How can you apply these types of communication skills to your everyday life? How can they be applied to communication with friends and family?

**Leadership Considerations:**
1. If a participant is not comfortable wearing a blindfold, the leader may allow him or her to close his or her eyes.
2. The leader may remind participants that they are allowed to slide hands along the rope. They are not required to hold the same area for the entire period.

3. The activity leader should ensure that the pair leader is giving proper and safe directions so that the blindfolded partner does not encounter any potential harm.

**Variations:**

1. The leader may choose to use abstract shapes versus geometric shapes.

2. The leader may allow participants to ask questions if unsure of the given directions.
3. To add difficulty to the task, the leader may choose three-dimensional shapes.

**Creator:** Theresa M. Connolly, CTRS, Illinois State University, Normal, Illinois.

# Cooperative Constructions

**Space Requirements:** Classroom or activity room

**Equipment/Resource Requirements:** Any odd or raw materials available (examples include old posters, string, tape, drinking straws, plastic silverware, old newspapers, cotton, and Popsicle sticks), instruction sheet (should be individually developed according to the materials available, see accompanying sample)

**Group Size:** Small group

**Program Goals:**
1. To increase participants' ability to follow directions.
2. To improve participants' ability to work cooperatively with peers.
3. To improve participants' problem-solving skills.

**Program Description:**
**Preparation:**
All materials should be grouped into piles with an equal amount of materials for each group. The leader will photocopy the appropriate number of instruction sheets, one for each group.

**Introduction:**
The leader will introduce the activity and explain that the purpose of the activity is to encourage the group to work cooperatively while creating an object that meets the requirements set by the leader.

**Activity Description:**
The leader should, depending on the group size, divide the participants into two to four equal groups. Next, the leader will hand out a copy of the instruction sheet to each group. The leader will explain that each group, while working cooperatively within the group, is to create an object, using the materials available, that meets the requirements outlined on the instruction sheet.

The groups should be given 25 to 30 minutes to create their constructions. Once all groups have completed their construction, the leader will discuss the following debriefing questions and focus on the goals of the activity.

**Debriefing Questions/Closure:**
1. What process did you use to create your construction?
2. Explain how it felt to have the group recognize and make use of your ideas.
3. Explain how it felt when the group did not recognize or make use of your ideas.
4. What techniques did your group use when individuals were in disagreement?
5. Describe any situations in your life when you needed to work cooperatively with others.
6. Explain how you would be able to apply the skills learned in this activity to your daily life activities.

**Leadership Considerations:**
1. The leader should ensure that all participants are contributing and that everyone's ideas are being heard.
2. The leader should walk around to make himself or herself available to answer any questions while the groups work.

**Variations:**
1. All groups can create an object related to a specific theme.
2. Each group's construction may focus on a specific area of leisure.
3. Each group can create criteria for the opposing group's constructions.

**Creator:** Theresa M. Connolly, CTRS, Illinois State University, Normal, Illinois.

# Cooperative Constructions

## Sample Instructions Sheet

Using the available materials, create an object which meets the requirements listed below:

- the object should have one handle;
- the object should have two holes;
- the object should be hollow;
- the object should have two structures connected to the inside;
- the object should have three structures connected to the outside;
- the object should have a rounded area;
- the object should have a squared area;
- the object should have one object piercing through the side;
- the object should be freestanding; and
- the object should have a moving part (such as a door or window).

# Are You Listening?

**Space Requirements:** Classroom or activity room

**Equipment/Resource Requirements:** Four different reading passages (appropriate level for the participants), paper, pencils, radio (if available), and blindfolds (one for each participant)

**Group Size:** Small group

**Program Goals:**
1. To increase participants' awareness of how interruptions affect the success of communication.
2. To increase participants' ability to block distractions and focus on what is being said.
3. To improve participants' ability to follow directions.

**Program Description:**
**Preparation:**
The leader should choose reading passages and collect all other materials prior to the start of the activity.

**Introduction:**
The leader will explain to the participants that this activity focuses on the ability to listen to others and to successfully block out those distractions that interfere with successful communication. The leader will explain that there will be several passages read to the participants.

**Activity Description:**
The leader will inform participants that they will be read a short passage or story and they need to listen carefully because it will be read only once. For the first passage, the leader will turn on the radio (or other noisy distraction) and begin reading the passage. The leader should not stop reading for any reason, regardless of the noise levels, distractions or interruptions. When the leader has finished reading, he or she will turn off the music and ask the participants to write down as much

as they can remember about the story. The leader will ask the participants to include as much detail as possible. The leader should give the participants a minimum of five minutes to recall and write details of the story.

Next, the leader will repeat the process of reading a story and the participants writing details implementing the following changes:

- Second time: have staff members come in and start up a side conversation.
- Third time: read passage under quiet situation.
- Fourth time: read story to participants with either their eyes closed or blindfolded.

Each passage that is read should be different in content. The leader will begin a discussion after all of the passages have been read.

For closure, the leader will ask participants to summarize the goals or purpose of this activity. The leader should use the debriefing questions to improve the participants' reflection of the purpose.

**Debriefing Questions/Closure:**
1. What did you write down or remember from each passage?
2. Which passage was the easiest for you to remember? Why?
3. What were some of the obstacles you had to overcome to hear and remember what was read?
4. For what reasons do you think we did this activity?
5. How many of you claim to be listening to others when in fact you are distracted or not listening at all?
6. How do you feel when others do not listen or remember what you said?
7. How do you think others feel when you do the same?

8. What can you do in the future to let others know or be aware that you are listening as they speak?

**Leadership Considerations:**
1. The leader should not reread any part of the passages.
2. The leader may change the number of passages read depending on amount of time available.

3. The leader should allow the participants to explain the story verbally if they are not comfortable with writing or are unable to write.
4. The leader should read passages that may relate to or interest the participants.

**Variations:**
1. The leader may have the participants watch television while he or she is reading the story.
2. The leader may have participants draw while he or she is reading the story.

**Creator:** Theresa M. Connolly, CTRS, Illinois State University, Normal, Illinois.

# Let's Work Together to Create a Volcano!

**Space Requirements:** Classroom or activity room.

**Equipment/Resource Requirements:** Two cardboard boxes, two empty juice cans, four cups of flour, two pitchers of water, four tablespoons of salt, one-half cup of baking soda, one cup vinegar, newspaper to cover the work surface, red food coloring, mixing bowls, mixing spoons, measuring spoons, measuring cup and dish soap

**Group Size:** Small group

**Program Goal:**
To increase participants' ability to cooperate in a small group activity.

**Program Description:**
   **Preparation:**
   Prior to the activity, the leader should have the newspapers spread across the working surface. The cardboard boxes also should be placed on the table; these are what the volcanoes will be built in. All other supplies should be set out, but not measured as the participants will be responsible for doing this.

   **Introduction:**
   The purpose of this activity is to promote cooperation within the group by building a volcano. The leader will begin by initiating a discussion on what it means to work cooperatively as part of a group. The leader can suggest some good group working techniques; for instance, sharing, taking turns, allowing everyone a chance to do something, not arguing. Participants may be asked to share their ideas.

   **Activity Description:**
   The first step in this activity is to build the volcano mold. This must dry overnight. The leader will divide the participants into two groups and give each group a cardboard box with a juice can in it. One person from each group will get the flour, pitcher of water, and salt. Each person in a group will take turns measuring the ingredients and pouring them into the mixing bowl. The water is a guessed aspect; if the mixture seems too thick, add more water. Each participant should take a turn stirring the mixture. Once the mixture is completely stirred, the participants may use their hands and mold the mixture around the juice can, completely covering the sides of the can.

   The volcano must dry overnight. The second step is to have the volcano erupt. A person from each group will get the food coloring, dish soap, baking soda, and vinegar. Next, a participant from each group will measure the ingredients and pour them into the juice can. The order for putting in the ingredients is: baking soda, dish soap, food coloring and, last, vinegar. Once the vinegar is placed in the juice can the volcano will erupt inside the box.

   The leader will end the activity by asking the participants to review which of the group techniques discussed earlier were used and which were not.

**Debriefing Questions/Closure:**
   1. How did it feel to work together in a group?
   2. Did you feel everyone received an equal chance to do part of the work?
   3. What are some of the things that make it difficult to work in a group? What makes it easy to work in a group?
   4. How did you go about dividing the tasks evenly?
   5. What are some advantages of working with others? What are some disadvantages?
   6. What did you learn from this activity that you can use in the future?

**Leadership Considerations:**
1. The leader should allow the participants to complete the project on their own, providing assistance only when necessary.
2. The leader should make sure all of the supplies are present. This project will not be successful without all of the supplies.

**Variations:**
1. The participants may do another activity, such as constructing something, that requires group cooperation.
2. The participants may do the activity as one large group.

**Creator:** Amy Conron, Illinois State University, Normal, Illinois.

# Describe Your Egg

**Space Requirements:** Classroom or activity room

**Equipment/Resource Requirements:** Hard-boiled eggs, egg coloring kit

**Group Size:** Small group

**Program Goals:**
1. To improve participants' ability to appreciate others' differences.
2. To improve participants' ability to appreciate their own differences.

**Program Description:**
**Preparation:**
Prior to the activity, the leader is responsible for boiling the eggs and gathering supplies.

**Introduction:**
The purpose of this activity is to increase participants' ability to follow directions and complete the designated task. The leader will ask participants to discuss the importance of being unique. Questions that may be used include:

- How are you like your best friend (or sister or brother)?
- How are you different from your best friend?
- Why is it important that you be unique from everyone else?
- Why is it important to tolerate other people's differences?

**Activity Description:**
To begin, the leader will give verbal directions and demonstrate to the group how to use the egg coloring kit. Next, the leader will distribute two or three eggs to each participant and allow the participants to color their eggs. The leader should encourage them to be creative in how they color their eggs.

After everyone has colored his or her eggs, the leader will gather the participants together for discussion and use the following questions.

**Debriefing Questions/Closure:**
1. Describe your eggs: colors, size, etc.
2. How are your eggs unique from the rest of the group's?
3. Like our eggs, how are we each unique from every other person in the group?
4. Why is it important to have unique characteristics?
5. Why is it important to recognize and appreciate people's differences?
6. How does this apply to your everyday life?

**Leadership Considerations:**
1. The leader should make sure that egg coloring is not ingested by anyone.
2. The leader should establish an atmosphere of acceptance.

**Variations:**
1. The participants may use clay figures instead of eggs.
2. Each participant may describe someone else's egg(s) in positive terms.

**Creator:** Connie Campbell, Illinois State University, Normal, Illinois.

# Who Is It?

**Space Requirements:** Classroom or activity room

**Equipment/Resource Requirements:** Blindfold

**Group Size:** Small group

**Program Goals:**
1. To increase participants' ability to exercise good listening skills.
2. To increase participants' ability to respond appropriately to conversational questions.
3. To improve participants' ability to give genuine compliments.

**Program Description:**
**Preparation:**
The leader will gather the equipment and instruct the participants to sit in a circle on the floor.

**Introduction:**
The leader will explain to the participants that they will be doing an activity that will require them to exercise good listening skills and appropriate social skills. Before starting the activity, all the participants in the group will introduce themselves, if they don't know each other.

**Activity Description:**
The leader will ask for a volunteer to be "it" first. This person will be blindfolded and seated in the center of the circle.

To begin, the leader will point to another individual in the group. This individual will say a positive statement; for example, "Hello, how are you?" Now, "it" must complete a series of steps in answering the question. To answer this correctly, "it" must say that individual's name, answer the question or respond appropriately to the

statement and say something positive about that particular person. If "it" does all the steps correctly, then the individual who spoke becomes "it."

If "it" does not complete all steps correctly, he or she continues to be "it" until he or she completes the steps correctly. To keep the activity challenging, it is recommended that all participants switch seats after a new individual becomes "it."

The leader will review the goals of the activity. The following questions may be used for closure.

**Debriefing Questions/Closure:**
1. How well did you remember everyone's name?
2. How easy or difficult was it to identify people by their voices?
3. How did you do coming up with answers to their questions?
4. How easy or difficult was it to give compliments? Receive compliments?
5. What lessons can be learned about communication skills?
6. How can you use what you learned today in the future?

**Leadership Consideration:**
The leader may go first so that he or she can demonstrate how to answer correctly.

**Variation:**
The participants may describe each other's favorite leisure activity or sports team.

**Creator:** Kate Czerwinski, Illinois State University, Normal, Illinois.

# Halloween Book

**Space Requirements:** Classroom or activity room

**Equipment/Resource Requirements:** Six pieces of construction paper per participant, crayons, stapler

**Group Size:** Small group

**Program Goals:**
1. To increase participants' ability to communicate through words and pictures.
2. To increase participants' ability to give and receive compliments.

**Program Description:**
**Preparation:**
The leader should prepare a completed example to show to the group.

**Introduction:**
The leader will explain to the participants that they will act as storybook writers for today's activity. They will be writing a Halloween story and drawing illustrations to go along with the story.

**Activity Description:**
The participants will sit at the table. The leader will explain to the group members that they each are to write a story that deals with Halloween and draw pictures that go along with the story. At this time, the leader may want to share the completed example with the group.

To get started, the leader will distribute six pieces of paper to each individual and encourage each individual to use all six pieces in his or her storybook construction. The leader will explain that it does not matter if the participants draw the pictures first or write the story, just as long as they do both. Once they have their story written, they should name their story and draw a cover for their book. Finally, the participants should staple the pages together so that it resembles a book. After all of the these steps are completed, each individual will read his or her story to the group.

The leader will ask the person to the reader's right to give the reader a compliment on some aspect of his or her book. The leader should make sure the reader responds appropriately.

The leader should close with a discussion focusing on the goals of the activity. Debriefing questions follow.

**Debriefing Questions/Closure:**
1. What did you try to communicate in your Halloween Book?
2. What is the major message or theme?
3. How did your illustrations help you communicate your ideas?
4. Did you draw the pictures or write the story line first?
5. Was it difficult creating a story?
6. What other things could you make a storybook about?
7. Do you like to be creative in ways like this? How about in other ways?

**Leadership Considerations:**
1. The leader should encourage all participants to be creative.
2. The leader should offer praise and acknowledge all individuals' stories and drawings.

**Variations:**
1. The leader may alter the content to reflect other upcoming holidays or leisure- and recreation-related activities.
2. Instead of individual storybooks, the participants can create one group book.

**Creator:** Jennifer Matkowich, Illinois State University, Normal, Illinois.

# Listening to New Ideas in Small Groups

**Space Requirements:** Classroom or activity room

**Equipment/Resource Requirements:** None

**Group Size:** Small group

**Program Goals:**
1. To increase participants' listening skills.
2. To increase participants' short-term memory skills.

**Program Description:**

**Preparation:**
The leader should prepare one or two sample stories.

**Introduction:**
The leader may introduce the activity as follows:

> Sometimes when working in a group, people aren't always listening to what others are saying and comprehending the ideas being stated. We may be thinking about what they are going to say next and not really listening to what is being said. Our activity for today will focus on carefully listening to others and improving listening skills.

**Activity Description:**
Everyone will sit in a circle. The leader will explain that the participants are going to play the game Telephone. The game will begin with the leader whispering a short story into the ear of the person next to him or her (without anyone else hearing). This person then will pass this story on as best as he or she can remember to the person next to him or her, and so on until everyone has heard the story. The last person to have heard the story will repeat the story aloud as accurately as he or she can remember. This story will be compared with the original story told by the leader.

This activity should be repeated a few times and different people should be allowed to create their own telephone story and be the leader.

The leader will conclude the activity by refocusing on the goals and discussing the following questions.

**Debriefing Questions/Closure:**
1. How different were the stories from the beginning to the end of the circle?
2. Why did the stories change?
3. Who do you need to go to if you want the original information or "the truth"?
4. What happens as stories are passed from one person to another?
5. How can you make sure that you have the information correctly when you repeat something?
6. What did you learn from this activity?
7. How will you use this information in the future?

**Leadership Consideration:**
The leader should remind participants that the person listening to the story may not ask any questions. He or she must repeat it exactly as he or she heard it.

**Variation:**
The participants may interview a partner to practice their listening skills. The leader should tell them that they will be responsible for remembering the information. The leader will have them report back to the group what their partner's answers were to the questions. Some example questions are favorite school subject, sport, food, or pet.

**Creator:** Amanda L. McGowen, Illinois State University, Normal, Illinois.

# Team Puzzle

**Space Requirements:** Classroom or activity room with table

**Equipment/Resource Requirements:** Accompanying illustrations cut into puzzles (one 10-piece puzzle for each participant, one envelope per puzzle)

**Group Size:** Small group

**Program Goals:**
1. To increase participants' ability to cooperate in groups.
2. To increase participants' positive conversation skills.
3. To increase participants' problem-solving ability.

**Program Description:**
**Preparation:**
The leader should use the accompanying work sheets for each puzzle or make up his or her own. The leader will cut each puzzle into ten pieces, mix up all of the pieces to all of the puzzles into one pile, and divide the pieces among the envelopes. The number of envelopes should depend on the number of participants.

**Introduction:**
The purpose of this activity is to have the participants work together to finish all the puzzles. While they are doing the puzzles they will be required to use positive conversation skills with one another.

Here is a suggestion for introducing the activity:

Today we are going to work together to finish [number of participants] puzzles. We need to use our please and thank yous. It is really important when working in a group to speak positively. You should say, "May I please have that piece," instead of, "Gimme that."

**Activity Description:**
The leader will explain to the group how important it is to work well in group situations and how important it is to use positive language. The leader will give examples of negative language and positive language and explain how the game will be played.

The leader will explain to the participants that they will each receive an envelope with puzzle pieces. The puzzle pieces belong to many different puzzles. The purpose of the activity is for all participants to work together to finish all of the puzzles. It is not important what puzzle gets done first, just that all the puzzles are finished. The participants have to help each other find the puzzle matches. While the participants work together, they are to only say positive things to each other.

The leader should give the participants ample time to complete the puzzles, and he or she should offer help where needed.

The leader should focus the group's attention on cooperation, conversational skills, and problem solving. Each is an important skill for the future. The following debriefing questions may help the group refocus on the goals.

**Debriefing Questions/Closure:**
1. Why is it important to work together?
2. Give an example of when cooperation really helped you.
3. Can someone give an example of positive language?
4. Why is positive language important?
5. Was it easy to cooperate when every puzzle needed to be finished?
6. Was it easy or difficult to work together?
7. What did you learn today during this activity that you can use this week?

**Leadership Considerations:**
1. The leader should continually remind participants to use positive language.
2. The leader should prepare puzzles that are appropriate for the age of the group members.

**Variations:**
1. The leader may add more puzzles to allow for a longer session.
2. The leader may choose to have the participants work together without speaking. They must exercise their nonverbal communication skills.
3. The participants may make their own puzzles.
4. The leader may create black and white puzzle pieces. After the puzzles are completed, the participants may color the puzzles.

**Creator:** Courtney Stauffer, Illinois State University, Normal, Illinois.

# Team Puzzle 1

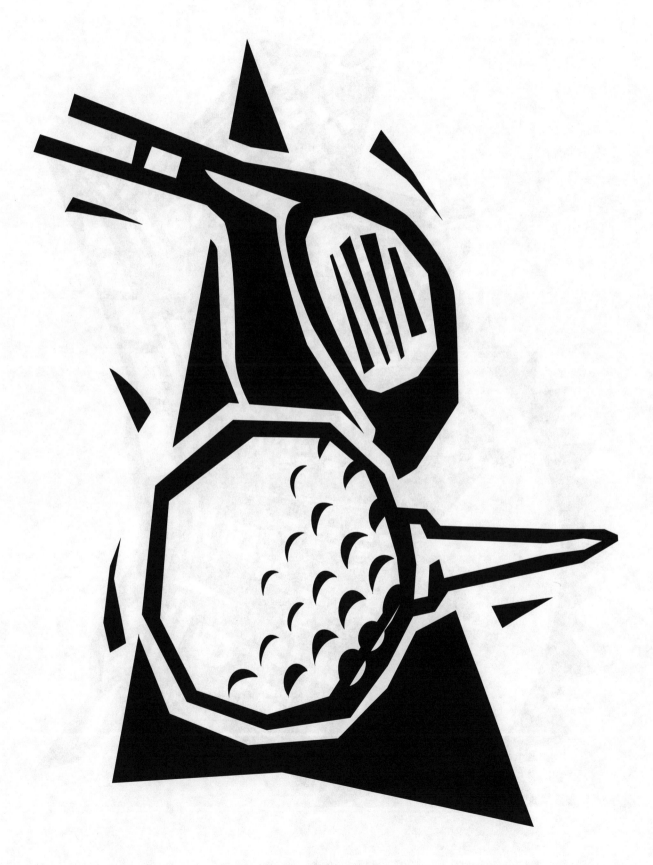

# Team Puzzle 2

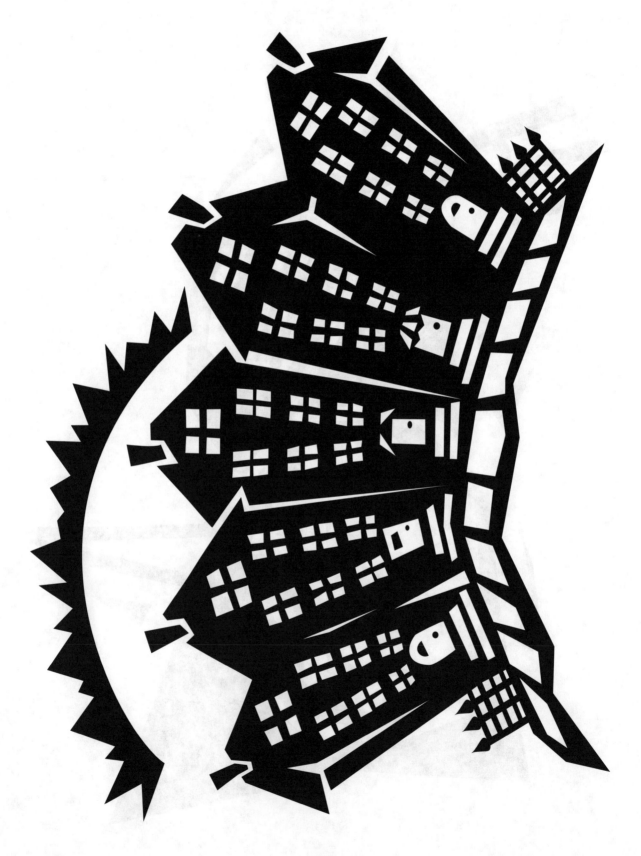

# Team Puzzle 3

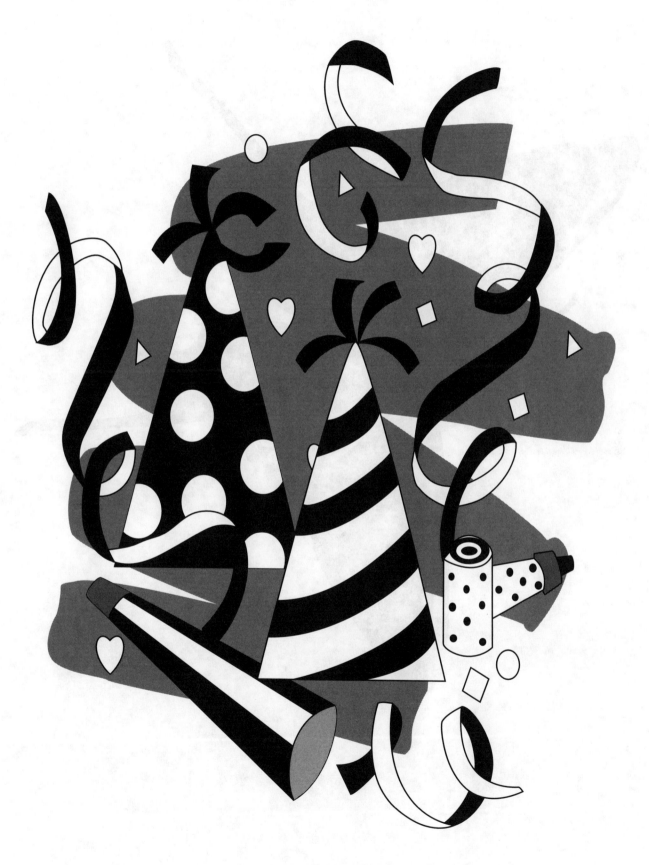

# Team Puzzle 4

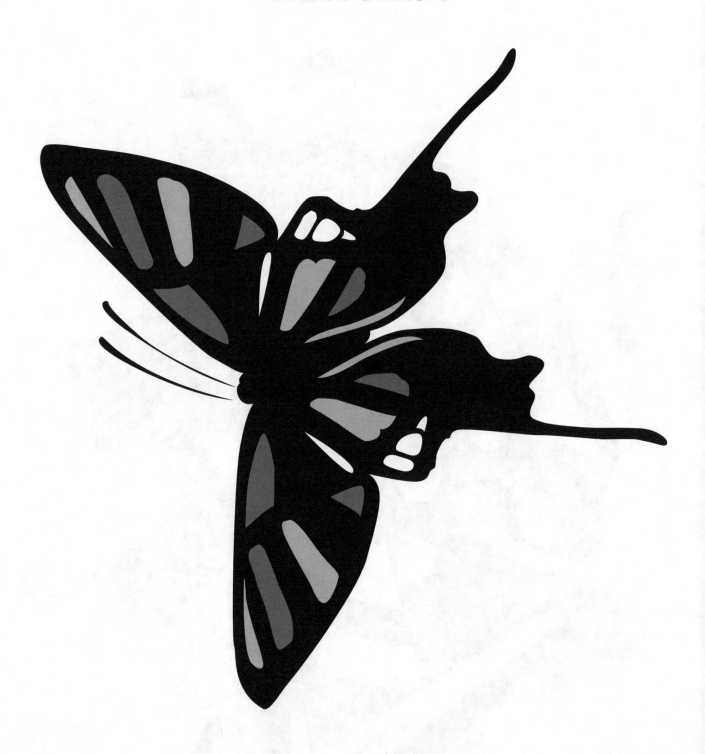

# Teamwork Egg Drop

**Space Requirements:** Classroom or activity room and a small area outside

**Equipment/Resource Requirements:** Eggs, cardboard, masking tape, toilet paper

**Group Size:** Small group

**Program Goals:**
1. To improve participants' ability to contribute to and work as a team member.
2. To improve participants' problem-solving ability.

**Program Description:**
**Preparation:**
Have the eggs, cardboard, tape, and toilet paper equally divided between the two teams.

**Introduction:**
The leader will divide the participants into two teams. The leader will explain to the group that they must work cooperatively with their teammates to construct a "carrier" for their egg to ride in. This carrier must protect the egg from breaking. The carrier will be dropped, with the egg inside, from various heights to see how high it can be dropped without breaking. The only rule for constructing the carrier is that each team must work as a group.

**Activity Description:**
The leader will distribute the materials to the groups and give them ample time to complete the carrier with the egg in it (the leader should set a time limit based on the overall time available). After each group has finished making its carrier, the groups will go outside. A staff member will drop each carrier from a high point (off playground equipment or table). After each car-

rier is dropped, it will be checked to see if the egg broke before it is dropped from a higher point.

The leader will end the activity by focusing on the goals of teamwork and problem solving. The leader will relate these two skills to everyday life and use the following debriefing questions to close the activity.

**Debriefing Questions/Closure:**
1. Ask each member of each group to share what his or her job was in preparing the structure.
2. Was the structure stronger due to the combining of everyone's ideas or was it weaker?
3. What were the benefits of working together as a group?
4. What did you take into consideration to solve the problem?
5. How were decisions made?
6. What did you learn from this activity?
7. How will you use what you have learned?

**Leadership Considerations:**
1. A staff member should drop the egg carrier to ensure the safety of the participants.
2. The leader should have the participants clean up any mess created from dropping the egg carrier.

**Variations:**
1. Each person may make a structure by himself or herself and drop it. Then they create one together as a group and compare which structure had a better chance of not breaking.
2. A water balloon may be used in place of an egg.

**Creator:** Amanda L. McGowen, Illinois State University, Normal, Illinois.

# Simon Senses

**Space Requirements:** Activity room or gymnasium

**Equipment/Resource Requirements:** Blindfolds

**Group Size:** Small group

**Program Goals:**
1. To increase participants' ability to follow directions and stay on task.
2. To increase participants' ability to give directions to a group.

**Program Description:**
**Preparation:**
The leader will prepare an open space—all tables and chairs should be cleared away. Each participant will put on a blindfold.

**Introduction:**
The purpose of the activity is to increase the participants' ability to follow directions by using sound. Another purpose of the activity is to allow the participants to lead a group.

The leader will open the activity with an introduction similar to the following:

> Who has played the game Simon Says before? This game is similar, it is called Simon Senses. You will not be able to use your eyes today—only your ears. It is really important that everyone listens well so you are able to hear all of the directions.
>
> Now it is time to put your blindfolds on so that we can get started. After I lead the activity, everyone in the group will get a chance to be Simon.

**Activity Description:**
The participants will form a line in front of the leader. The leader is Simon. The leader will call the directions for the participants to move.

Like in Simon Says, the participants should only move at certain times. The game will be played by sound. Each participant, except the leader, will wear a blindfold. The leader will call out directions. The participants will have to listen carefully.

After the leader has led the game a couple of times, each participant will be given the opportunity to be Simon and lead. The activity is finished when everyone has led at least once. Participants do not wear a blindfold when they lead.

The leader will summarize the activity by restating the goals and emphasizing the debriefing questions.

**Debriefing Questions/Closure:**
1. How important is it to listen to directions?
2. What happens when you don't listen well?
3. Who likes leading games or activities? Why?
4. Who thinks they gave good directions?
5. What makes directions easy to follow?
6. What did you learn during this activity?

**Leadership Considerations:**
1. The leader should make sure blindfolds are the appropriate size for the group.
2. When the participants lead, the leader should tell them ahead of time that the directions have to be appropriate and fair.

**Variation:**
The participants may play by only using their eyes and no verbal directions. They may exchange the "Simon says" with a clap.

**Creator:** Courtney Stauffer, Illinois State University, Normal, Illinois.

# What Are They Feeling?

**Space Requirements:** Classroom or activity room

**Equipment/Resource Requirements:** 3-by-5-inch index cards, marker

**Group Size:** Small group

**Program Goals:**
1. To improve participants' ability to recognize nonverbal communication.
2. To improve participants' ability to display nonverbal communication.

**Program Description:**
**Preparation:**
The leader should prepare a space for teams to act out situations. The leader should make up game cards in advance. Possible situations for the game cards include:

- excited children at a circus;
- waking up in the morning feeling tired;
- a bored student listening to a lecture;
- the meeting of two friends who begin to have an argument;
- a child consoling a sad friend;
- a parent angrily scolding her apologetic child for breaking a glass;
- two friends walking up to a door that has something scary behind it;
- an anxious parent waiting for a child, who is late, to return home;
- getting a lower grade than what you expected;
- doing a good deed for someone you don't know well;
- opening a birthday gift;
- waiting for the school bus to come down the road;
- bandaging a friend's injured knee;
- receiving a compliment for doing something well;
- winning an award for doing something well;
- giving a book report when you're not prepared;
- a bicyclist speeds by, almost knocking you over; and
- a small child watching a scary movie.

**Introduction:**
The purpose of this activity is to help participants increase their knowledge of nonverbal communication.

A suggestion for introducing the activity is as follows:

> What are some different types of nonverbal communication? Do people sometimes have nonverbal communication that doesn't match their verbal communication? Which type do you believe?

Next, the leader will divide the group into two teams to act out all the situations. When one group is acting, the other group will be guessing. After a participant picks a card, his or her team will go to a spot where the other team will not be able to hear. The team members will discuss how they will act out the activity on the card.

**Activity Description:**
The leader will have game cards ready to play. The leader will explain that participants will pick out a game card and act it out as a team. The other group guesses what they are acting. The leader should allow each group to act one card each turn. The leader should offer help where needed to act out the situation.

When all the cards have been acted or time is up, the participants will name four emotions that were acted out. The leader and the participants will discuss the different types of emotions and how nonverbal communication helps express those emotions.

The leader will refocus the group on the goals of recognizing and displaying nonverbal communication. The participants will apply what they've learned to their future. The leader will use the debriefing questions.

**Debriefing Questions/Closure:**
1. What are some positive nonverbal communication techniques?
2. What are some negative nonverbal communication techniques?
3. What happens when verbal communication doesn't match the nonverbal communication?
4. What do people think when you are showing negative nonverbal communication?
5. What do people think when you are showing positive nonverbal communication?
6. How can you use what you've learned today?

**Leadership Considerations:**
1. The leader should make sure each participant is involved within the group.
2. The leader should offer assistance if an extra person is needed to act in a situation.

**Variations:**
1. The participants may act out individually and not in groups.
2. The leader may change the game cards according to the needs of the group.

**Creator:** Courtney Stauffer, Illinois State University, Normal, Illinois.

# Put Teamwork to the Test

**Space Requirements:** Gymnasium

**Equipment/Resource Requirements:** Blindfolds, paper cups, scarves, beachballs, objects to use as obstacles

**Group Size:** Small group

**Program Goals:**
1. To increase participants' ability to work together.
2. To increase participants' ability to speak positively.

**Program Description:**

**Preparation:**
The leader will prepare the gym for different teamwork activities. The leader will spread the obstacles throughout one half of the gym, leaving an open path around the outside of the gym.

**Introduction:**
The purpose of this activity is to allow participants to improve teamwork and cooperation skills while using positive conversation skills.

A suggestion for introducing the activity is as follows:

Today we are going to put our teamwork to the test with a Teamwork Olympics. Everyone needs to accept who his or her partner is and work well with him or her.

**Activity Description:**
The leader will pair up the participants. The leader will explain the rules and the order of the events. There are no winners. The purpose is for every team to finish each event.

*First Event—The Three-Legged Race:*
The participants stand side-by-side and tie a scarf around their inside legs. Now they will have to walk around the gym three times with three legs.

*Second Event—Beachball Bellies:* The participants face each other. A beachball is placed between their stomachs. They have to walk around the gym twice without the beachball falling. *They must not use their hands!*

*Third Event—Guide Your Partner:* Obstacles have been put on the floor. One partner is blindfolded and the other is a guide. The guide has to guide his or her partner through the obstacle course.

*Fourth Event—Paper Cup Towers:* Each pair of participants is given a stack of cups with which to build a tower. The participants are trying to build the tallest tower. They must use all the cups given to them.

After all events are completed, the group will discuss the concept of teamwork.

**Debriefing Questions/Closure:**
1. Why is teamwork important?
2. Describe a situation where teamwork has played an important part in your success.
3. Were these games difficult to do? Could you have done them by yourself?
4. What happens if you're not happy with your partner? Should that affect your teamwork?
5. Where in life would teamwork be useful?
6. How can you use what you learned today in the future?

**Leadership Considerations:**
1. The leader should pair participants who are close in height.

2. The leader should make sure everyone is doing the events on task.
3. The leader should decide how many times the participants are to go around the gym based on their abilities.

**Variations:**
1. The leader may have the participants come up with additional teamwork activities.

2. The participants may compete for points.
3. The participants may be teamed up with staff members.

**Creator:** Courtney Stauffer, Illinois State University, Normal, Illinois.

# My Emotional Poem

**Space Requirements:** Classroom or activity room

**Equipment/Resource Requirements:** Paper, pencils, tape player, music tape

**Group Size:** Small group

**Program Goals:**
1. To increase participants' ability to communicate or express emotions.
2. To allow participants the opportunity to express creativity through poem writing.

**Program Description:**
**Preparation:**
The leader should locate a music tape, preferably instrumental music. Also, a completed example of a poem should be available to share with the group. The leader should place supplies on the table.

**Introduction:**
The leader should explain to the participants that they will be doing an activity that requires them to be creative in expressing their emotions. At this time, it may be necessary to hold a discussion on emotions, what they are, when they happen, and examples of emotions.

**Activity Description:**
The leader will begin the activity by having participants either sit or lie on the floor. Next, the leader will play the music tape. It is recommended that the tape consist of instrumental music only. The leader will instruct the participants to close their eyes while listening to the music and try to visualize what the music is about. After a few minutes, the leader will ask the participants the following questions. This should be done with the music playing softly in the background. Also, participants' eyes should remain closed during this time.

1. What does the music make you think about?
2. What colors do you see?
3. What time of the year is it?
4. What kinds of places do you see?
5. Do you see mountains? Water?

After discussing the preceding questions, the leader will explain to the participants that they are now going to individually write a poem. The content of the poem should relate to the music and any emotions that were stirred or felt while listening to the music. The leader should encourage the participants to add pictures and/or whatever else would be helpful in describing their reaction to the music.

The leader should explain that the poem can, but does not have to, rhyme. The participants are free to write it however they wish. At this time the leader should show an example to the group and distribute one piece of paper and writing utensil to each person.

The leader should give the group an example of how to start a poem, for instance, "I hear music, I see _____. I feel _____. It reminds me of _____." Each group participant can start the poem like this or in his or her own unique way. It is recommended that the music continue to be played during this time.

The leader should give the participants 25–30 minutes working time. Next, each participant will share his or her poem with the group. The leader will conclude the session by discussing the following questions.

**Debriefing Questions/Closure:**
1. What emotions did you feel while the music played?
2. How does music help us express our emotions?
3. How did writing a poem help you express emotions?

4. Was it easy or difficult for you to be creative in writing a poem?
5. Why is it important to find constructive ways to express emotions?

**Leadership Consideration:**
The leader should tell everyone to be respectful while others are reading their poems aloud.

**Variation:**
The leader may have the group work together to write one poem.

**Creator:** Lazheta Thomas, Illinois State University, Normal, Illinois.

# A Puppet's Rights

**Space Requirements:** Classroom or activity room

**Equipment/Resource Requirements:** Paper bags, construction paper, yarn, markers, fabric scraps, glue, scissors, deck of cards with scenarios illustrating standing up for and not standing up for individual rights (see the examples)

**Group Size:** Small group

**Program Goals:**
1. To increase participants' knowledge of personal rights.
2. To improve participants' ability to verbalize their own individual personal rights.
3. To improve participants' communication techniques in relation to personal rights.

**Program Description:**
**Preparation:**
The leader should have paper bags and supplies set out for participants ahead of time. Sample scenarios include:

- someone uses your property without permission;
- you want to go to sleep and your roommate wants the light on;
- you want to go to the library on Saturday and no one else does;
- you get up from the couch and someone takes your spot; and
- a visitor is sitting on your bed.

**Introduction:**
The purpose of this activity is to provide participants with the opportunity to increase knowledge of their personal rights, and their ability to verbalize their own rights, while developing techniques to communicate these rights effectively to others.

**Activity Description:**
The leader should state the goals of the activity, and then hold a discussion on what personal rights are and participants' own individual rights.

The leader will give instructions for the activity. The participants will make a puppet out of the paper bags. The leader will tell the participants that these puppets will be used in a mini puppet show with a partner.

After the puppets are made, the leader will give instructions for the second part of the activity. Participants will select situation cards to be acted out with their puppet and a partner's puppet. The leader will allow two to three minutes per scenario. The leader will discuss each scenario and involve all participants. The leader will restate the goals and purpose of the activity.

**Debriefing Questions/Closure:**
1. What are personal rights?
2. What are your personal rights?
3. In what situation have your personal rights been invaded?
4. How did you handle the situation?
5. How could you handle situations in the future?
6. What have you learned about personal rights?

**Leadership Considerations:**
1. The leader should encourage participants to be creative and give their puppet a name.
2. The leader should encourage participants to act out the situation in the best possible way to get the most positive results.
3. The leader should tell participants that sticking up for their rights does not mean encouraging a fight, but means expressing one's rights in a positive way in order to prevent further problems.

4. The leader should encourage participants to think back to what their puppet would say if they ever felt they may not be able to stand up for their rights.

**Variations:**

1. The participants can create a body puppet character out of paper grocery bags.

2. Older participants can role-play and work on decision-making skills when problems with peer pressure arise.

**Creator:** Renee Raczkowski, Illinois State University, Normal, Illinois.

# Circular Art

**Space Requirements:** Classroom or activity room

**Equipment/Resource Requirements:** Construction paper, pencils, markers or crayons, radio or tape player (music tape)

**Group Size:** Small group

**Program Goals:**
1. To increase participants' ability to follow directions and remain on task.
2. To increase participants' ability to cooperate with a group to create an art project.

**Program Description:**
**Preparation:**
The leader should gather the materials.

**Introduction:**
The leader will introduce the activity and give an overview of the directions.

**Activity Description:**
The leader will distribute one sheet of paper and a drawing utensil to each participant. The leader should place the markers or crayons on the table, within reach of all group members.

The leader will begin by instructing everyone to put his or her first and last name in the upper right-hand corner of the piece of paper. After this is done, the leader will explain to the participants that it is now time to use their creativity. When the music starts they should draw, write or do whatever they choose on their piece of paper. When they hear the music stop, they should stop what they are doing and put their marker or crayon down.

At this point, the leader will give the group a direction to follow, for example: pass papers to the right, pass papers to the left, pass papers to the person sitting across the table, or pass papers to the person sitting two seats to the left. The next person continues drawing on the new sheet, with each person drawing something on each other person's sheet of paper. Directions should continue until all papers are back in front of the original owners.

After the pictures are drawn, each person will take a turn telling the group a story about his or her picture or paper. He or she can tell the group what the picture reminds him or her of or he or she can make up an interesting, creative story. The leader should conclude the activity by discussing the following questions.

**Debriefing Questions/Closure:**
1. Was it difficult or easy to be creative in your drawing?
2. How did you feel about passing your paper around and allowing everyone to see and add to your drawing?
3. What did you think of the end result of your art work? Were you able to recognize it?
4. How did cooperation of other group members change your picture?

**Leadership Considerations:**
1. The leader should tell the group to respect everyone's picture and not to criticize anyone's work.
2. The leader should tell the participants not to scribble on top of someone else's work.
3. The leader should encourage the participants to be positive in their drawings.

**Variation:**
The leader may give the group a theme to draw, i.e., leisure activities or leisure resources.

**Creator:** Lazheta Thomas, Illinois State University, Normal, Illinois.

# Cooperative Win, Lose, or Mold

**Space Requirements:** Classroom or activity room

**Equipment/Resource Requirements:** Play-Doh

**Group Size:** Small group

**Program Goals:**
1. To improve participants' ability to cooperate as a means of reaching a common goal.
2. To increase participants' communication skills with others in a group.
3. To increase participants' ability to compromise and make decisions as a group.

**Program Description:**
**Preparation:**
The leader should prepare a list of objects to be molded ahead of time. The leader will purchase different colors of Play-Doh.

**Introduction:**
The purpose of this activity is to improve cooperation, communication, and compromise skills, while working together to achieve a common goal.

**Activity Description:**
The leader should state the goals and purpose of the activity. The leader will open with a discussion on appropriate cooperative, communication and compromise skills necessary for working together.

The leader should give instructions for the activity. The participants get into two teams or select a partner (depending on size of group). Each team will be given a can of Play-Doh. The leader will state an object to be molded. Each group or set of partners must work together and each person must mold a part of the object stated.

The first group to make the object, raise their hands, and show it to the leader, will receive a point. The team or pair with the most points at the end of the game will receive a prize. The leader will direct a discussion on problems participants faced, and what could have been done better. Also, the leader will discuss how communication skills are necessary in everyday life.

The leader will close and restate the goals of the activity.

**Debriefing Questions/Closure:**
1. How did you communicate with the group or with your partner?
2. What problems did you face while participating in the activity?
3. How did you handle these difficulties?
4. What could have been done to make the activity run more smoothly?
5. In what way did you compromise to reach the final product?
6. Give a situation in everyday life where we all need to cooperate. Give a situation in everyday life where we all need to communicate. Give a situation in everyday life where we all need to compromise.

**Leadership Considerations:**
1. The leader will give an example of how the activity will work.
2. The leader will tell the participants that each person must contribute or his or her team will not receive a point.
3. The leader will encourage participants to communicate effectively with their group by stating which part they will make.

**Variations:**
1. This activity can be implemented to incorporate increasing knowledge of leisure resources or leisure activities.
2. Competition can be downplayed with each group or set of partners receiving points for creativity in molding the object.

**Creator:** Renee Raczkowski, Illinois State University, Normal, Illinois.

# Story Libs

**Space Requirements:** Classroom or activity room

**Equipment/Resource Requirements:** Well-known story or nursery rhyme, such as "Mary Had a Little Lamb," with certain words omitted

**Group Size:** Small group

**Program Goal:**
To increase participants' ability to cooperate as a means of reaching a common goal.

**Program Description:**
**Preparation:**
The leader will choose a story and prepare it ahead of time (see the example).

**Introduction:**
The purpose of this activity is to provide the opportunity for participants to increase cooperation skills.

**Activity Description:**
The leader begins by stating the goals and purpose of the activity. The leader will allow a brief discussion on cooperation skills in relation to everyday activities.

The leader should give instructions for the activity. Participants will be asked to contribute a word when asked by the leader, for example, "What is a girl's name?"

The leader will continue to go around the circle asking the participants to contribute a word. The words that are collected will be written down by the leader, in the blank areas in a story. A silly story will be created from the words the participants contributed. The leader will read the story aloud. The leader will hold a discussion on the importance of working together and restate the goals of the activity, using the following debriefing questions for closure.

**Debriefing Questions/Closure:**
1. What are the reasons why it is important to work together?
2. In what other situations is it important to work together?
3. Explain the saying, "Two heads are better than one."

**Leadership Considerations:**
1. The leader will allow the participants to "pass" if they want to.
2. The leader will assist participants with ideas if appropriate.
3. The leader will encourage participants to speak only when it is their turn.

**Variations:**
1. This activity may be implemented for a participant to work on his or her own. The leader should give him or her a work sheet with a list of words that are numbered. Then the leader will have him or her place the words into the story with the corresponding numbers.
2. If the participants can write, the leader may ask them to write their responses. The leader should go around the circle and allow them to read their responses. The leader may want to go around again to create a different story.

**Creator:** Renee Raczkowski, Illinois State University, Normal, Illinois.

# Story Libs

Example of original story:

Mary had a little lamb whose fleece was white as snow. Everywhere that Mary went, the lamb was sure to go.

Example of story with blanks:

  1   had a little   2   whose fleece was white as   3  . Everywhere that   4   went, the   5   was sure to go.

   1. Girl's name            _____
   2. Animal                  _____
   3. Weather condition    _____
   4. Girl's name            _____
   5. Animal                  _____

# Listen in the Jungle

**Space Requirements:** Classroom or activity room

**Equipment/Resource Requirements:** Ropes, Hula-Hoops, boxes, other obstacles

**Group Size:** Small group

**Program Goals:**
1. To improve participants' listening skills.
2. To increase participants' ability to follow directions.

**Program Description:**
**Preparation:**
The leader should set up the obstacle course ahead of time.

**Introduction:**
This activity is designed to help individuals learn to work as a team. This activity requires decision-making, cooperation, and good listening skills.

**Activity Description:**
The leader should design an obstacle course either easy or difficult depending on the skill level of the participants. The leader will begin by explaining the directions of the activity to the group. This should take place in a room where the obstacle course is *not* set up. The leader should not let any group members see the obstacle course.

The leader will explain to the participants that they are to pretend that they are deep in the jungle. It is nighttime and there is only one person who has special powers to see in the dark. At this time, the leader will inform the participants (as a group) to choose one person who will have the special power of night vision. This person will be responsible for getting all of his or her group members across the jungle safely. This will require accurate and precise verbal directions to be given and patience to be exercised by the entire group.

After a night-vision leader has been chosen, it is time to distribute one blindfold to each group member (except for the person with special night-vision powers). The group members will get in line, hold hands or shoulders, and be led into the obstacle area. The first person in line, or the first volunteer, will be the first person who will cross the jungle.

At this point, the night-vision leader gives verbal directions to the blindfolded person, explaining in the best possible detail how to avoid the obstacles. If at any time during the crossing an obstacle is touched, the participant must immediately lie down and become an obstacle for the participants yet to cross.

The night-vision leader may direct the individuals by using instructions such as go right, take two steps to the left, duck down, step over. After the first person crosses, play continues until all participants have had a turn.

The challenge increases after the first person completes the course. When the second person crosses the course, the rules of the night-vision leader are modified. Instead of saying, "Duck down," a clap will indicate the phrase. When the third person crosses the course, a "beep" sound replaces the phrase, "Step over." These replacement sounds must be used for the rest of the participants also.

Once all group members have safely crossed the course, the night-vision leader must blindfold himself or herself and cross the course from memory. The only assistance that can be given to that individual is the replies of yes or no from the other participants, who will no longer be wearing blindfolds.

When there are only five minutes left in the period, the group leader will stop the activity, review the purpose of the activity (listening skills, decision-making skills, and cooperation), and discuss the following questions.

**Debriefing Questions/Closure:**
1. Why was it important to work as a team in this activity?
2. What things could you have done to work better as a team?
3. Was the activity easier when you could hear the leader?
4. What could you have done to make things easier on yourself and your team?

**Leadership Considerations:**
1. The leader should explain that the participants could trip on an obstacle and get hurt during the activity, so they should be sure to carefully listen to all directions.
2. The leader should explain that the night-vision leader may only talk each participant through the course, and may not touch the individual.
3. The leader should decide ahead of time whether participants will be allowed to ask questions while crossing the obstacle course.

**Variation:**
The leader can decrease the challenge by having the participants step out of the course when they touch an obstacle on the course, rather than lying down on the course and becoming an obstacle.

**Creator:** Jessica Kamm, Illinois State University, Normal, Illinois.

# Cooperation Murals

**Space Requirements:** Classroom or activity room

**Equipment/Resource Requirements:** Crayons, markers or colored pencils, large precut paper squares, rope or string

**Group Size:** Small group

**Program Goals:**
1. To improve participants' ability to cooperate with a peer.
2. To improve participants' ability to compromise with a peer.

**Program Description:**
**Preparation:**
The leader will prepare one large precut square for every two participants. The leader will gather other supplies.

**Introduction:**
The purpose of this activity is to provide participants with an opportunity to engage in a cooperative partner activity while utilizing proper techniques of respect, patience and compromise.

**Activity Description:**
The leader should state the goals and purpose of the activity. The leader will instruct all participants to find a partner who they will be able to work well with or the leader may assign partners. The participants then will have their hands tied to their partners' hands. For example, one partner's right hand will be tied to the other partner's left hand. Materials will be distributed and the participants will be instructed to draw a picture with their partner, using the previously discussed skills of patience, compromise and respect.

After the pictures are completed the participants will have an opportunity to talk both individually and as a pair. The leader will restate the goals and purpose of the activity and allow the group members to comment about what they learned.

**Debriefing Questions/Closure:**
1. Why is compromise important?
2. In what everyday situations do we need to compromise?
3. What does it take to be patient?
4. What is involved in cooperation?
5. How did you handle your partner's frustration?
6. What did you learn about cooperation, compromise, and patience?

**Leadership Considerations:**
1. The leader should be sensitive about tying wrists. The leader should know the backgrounds of his or her participants.
2. As an alternative to tying, a cotton ball may be placed between the back of the partners' hands and the partners are advised not to let it drop.

**Variations:**
1. The leader may give the partners a theme for their drawing.
2. The leader may specify additional rules, such as using nondominant hands.

**Creator:** Monika Ressel, Illinois State University, Normal, Illinois.

# Problem-Solving, Decision-Making, and Planning Skills

# Crack the Code

**Space Requirements:** Outside or throughout building

**Equipment/Resource Requirements:** Clue cards, accompanying form as decoder, pens and pencils

**Group Size:** Small group

**Program Goals:**
1. To increase participants' group cooperation skills.
2. To increase participants' problem-solving skills.

**Program Description:**

**Preparation:**
The leader must prepare clue cards in special code and place them in designated locations prior to this activity. Preparation is the key for success in this activity. This is essentially a scavenger hunt. The clue cards have to be written in special code (see accompanying form). Different sites must be chosen and each clue should lead to the next site (e.g., Clue: Where could you get a drink? Next location: Drinking fountain).

**Introduction:**
The purpose of the activity is to increase participants' group cooperation skills and problem-solving skills.

A suggestion for introducing the activity is as follows:

We are going to go on a scavenger hunt. This is not the usual scavenger hunt, this one is in secret code. You have to work with your partners to crack the code.

**Activity Description:**
The leader will divide the participants into two teams. Each participant will receive a copy of the decoder card. The leader will give the participants the first clue to decode and let them go from there. There are no winner and losers. Each team is encouraged to finish.

After the teams have found all the clues and returned, they will sit in a circle to discuss the activity. The leader will focus the discussion on the goals of cooperation and problem-solving skills.

**Debriefing Questions/Closure:**
1. How did you crack the codes?
2. Why was it important to work together?
3. Were the clues difficult to solve?
4. What problems did you encounter?
5. How essential was cooperation to your team's success?
6. How did your group go about seeing where the next clue would be?
7. Describe a situation this week that will require cooperation and problem-solving skills.

**Leadership Considerations:**
1. The leader will encourage everyone to finish.
2. The leader may have a staff member go with each group.

**Variations:**
1. Individuals may play for themselves instead of on teams.
2. The participants may map out the facility.
3. The participants may plan the whole hunt.

**Creator:** Courtney Stauffer, Illinois State University, Normal, Illinois.

# Crack the Code

| | | | | | |
|---|---|---|---|---|---|
| A | B | C | D | E | F |
| G | H | I | J | K | L |
| M | N | O | P | Q | R |
| S | T | U | V | W | X |
| | | Y | Z | | |

# Footprints

**Space Requirements:** Arts and crafts room with water readily available

**Equipment/Resource Requirements:** Medium-sized tub or dishpan (optional), various colors of tempera paint (optional), white drawing paper, accompanying work sheet, pencils, paper towels, newspapers, glue, and markers

**Group Size:** Small group

**Program Goals:**
1. To increase participants' awareness of decisions made in the past.
2. To increase participants' ability to identify future goals.
3. To increase participants' ability to assume responsibility for decisions made in the past, present, and future.

**Program Description:**
**Preparation:**
Prior to the start of the activity, the leader will have all materials prepared and ready for use. This includes preparing two or three medium sized tubs or dishpans by pouring a thin layer of tempera paint into each and setting the tubs of paint on the floor on top of old newspapers.

**Introduction:**
The purpose of this activity is to encourage participants to share past decisions and future goals while they learn the skills necessary to assume responsibility for future decisions.

**Activity Description:**
The leader will begin the activity by explaining to participants that they will be making footprints with tempera paint onto a sheet of drawing paper. Prior to making footprints, the participants will wash their feet.

Then the leader will have each participant write his or her name somewhere on his or her piece of paper so he or she can later identify which prints belong to him or her. Next, the participants will take turns placing one or both feet into the paint and then making several footprints onto the outer edges of their paper, leaving room in the center of the page. Once this is done, the participants will wash the paint off of their feet.

Once the group has completed prints, the leader will distribute one Footprints work sheet to each individual (see accompanying form). Participants should be given approximately 20 minutes to complete the work sheet. Once work sheets have been completed, the leader will ask all participants to glue their work sheet to the center of the drawing paper, between their footprints. The leader will use the work sheet for debriefing questions.

**Debriefing Questions/Closure:**
See questions on accompanying Footprints work sheet.

**Leadership Considerations:**
1. If participants do not wish to place feet in paint, they may use hands.
2. The leader should have the participants look at footprints as they complete the work sheet.
3. The leader should make sure paint is completely dry before allowing participants to take activity home.
4. The leader may choose to have the participants outline their feet or hands versus placing their hands or feet in paint.
5. The leader will use the work sheet as a debriefing tool.

**Variations:**
1. The leader may choose to create a bulletin board out of footprints with questions in center of board.

2.  The leader may choose to use hand prints and change questions to deal with what hands have done in the past and what hands will do in the future.

3.  The leader may choose to use lipstick and have participants kiss the paper. Questions would then deal with what participants have said in the past and what will be said in the future.

**Creator:** Theresa M. Connolly, CTRS, Illinois State University, Normal, Illinois.

# Footprints

Please answer the following questions as completely and with as much detail as possible.

1. Where have these feet been?

2. Where are these feet now?

3. How did these feet get here?

4. Where are these feet going?

5. How will these feet get to where they are going?

6. What kind of help will these feet need to get where they are going?

7. Write three goals for the future of these feet.

# Shopping for Value

**Space Requirements:** Grocery store

**Equipment/Resource Requirements:** List of items to find

**Group Size:** Small group (two or three children)

**Program Goals:**
1. To increase participants' ability to compare prices of goods.
2. To increase participants' ability to make purchasing decisions based on price and value.

**Program Description:**
**Preparation:**
The leader will prepare a list of items to be obtained during the trip before the activity meeting.

**Introduction:**
The leader will introduce the idea of prices on items, and the concept of value, e.g., lowest price is not always the best value.

**Activity Description:**
The leader will take a small group of children (two or three) to a grocery store. Each participant will receive a list of items that will be compared at the grocery store. The leader will explain to them that they are to find the item for the lowest cost; for example, there may be a can of soup on the list and the store brand is priced less compared to the national brand name. They need to choose the soup with the lowest price and then decide if it's the best value.

The leader will have the group look at different items, such as candy, soda, snacks, and produce. If possible, the leader will purchase items that they can eat later. This activity may be a good time to discuss price value as well as nutritional and energy value.

The leader will close the session with a discussion of the activity goals and review the debriefing questions.

**Debriefing Questions/Closure:**
1. If we look at two products, how do we know which is the less expensive?
2. How do we determine which product has the best price value? How do we determine which product has the best overall value?
3. How do we make these decisions?
4. Why are we concerned about the price and value of what we buy?

**Leadership Considerations:**
1. The leader will make sure there is supervision at the store in order to avoid problems.
2. The grocery store should be contacted ahead of time by the leader for permission to conduct this activity.
3. Research is required on behalf of the leader prior to the activity to determine the least expensive prices for particular items.

**Variations:**
1. If the participants are older and able to demonstrate an increased level of responsibility, the leader may allow them to have money to actually pay for the items.
2. Also, if the group consists of adolescents or teens, the leader may have the participants spend their own money.
3. The group may go to another type of store, e.g., department store, and shop for leisure equipment.
4. The leader may have the participants use the same idea to determine what to do on a weekend day or night trip.

**Creator:** Kristen Boys, Illinois State University, Normal, Illinois.

# Community Leisure Resource Relay

**Space Requirements:** Gymnasium or large playing area

**Equipment/Resource Requirements:** Footballs, baseballs, baseball gloves, paper grocery bags, markers, assorted pamphlets and informative brochures from area community agencies

**Group Size:** Small group

**Program Goals:**
1. To increase participants' awareness of community resources.
2. To increase participants' ability to work with others.
3. To allow participants the opportunity to plan a trip to one community agency.

**Program Description:**
**Preparation:**
Prior to implementing the activity, the leader should gather a variety of informative brochures and pamphlets from local community leisure- and recreation-related agencies. It will be necessary to collect two copies of each resource to play the game.

In setting up the game, the leader should take each paper bag and label it with a category and a number (see examples). The names and numbers will vary depending on the number of supplies and resources collected. Some examples of categories are as follows:

1. YWCA and YMCA
2. Bloomington/Normal Park Departments
3. Sports Equipment
4. The Discovery Museum
5. Jumping Jack's
6. Miller Park Zoo

During the game there will be two teams, therefore there should be two sets of bags labeled exactly the same. Also, the resources and equip-

ment should be identical. Before the activity begins, the leader should place both sets of bags at one end of the activity area. The resource information and the equipment should be placed at the opposite end of the activity area, one pile for each team.

**Introduction:**
The purpose of this activity is to increase participants' awareness of community leisure and recreation resources, increase their ability to work with others as part of a team, and allow participants the opportunity to help plan their own trip to a community agency.

A suggested way for introducing the activity is as follows:

Today we are going to focus on some resources that can be found within the community. These resources will be helpful to you in planning your community out-trip. They will help you identify some of the choices or options that are available to you.

**Activity Description:**
The leader will begin the activity by dividing the group into two teams and lining them up behind each pile of resources and equipment. On the leader's command, a team member from each team must run to his or her team's pile, grab a resource or piece of equipment and then run to his or her team's set of grocery bags. The object of the activity is to place the resources and equipment into the bag that represents the most suitable category for that particular item. Each participant is allowed to take one item at a time to the bags.

The game will end when all of the items have been placed into the bags. At the conclusion of the activity, the leader and the groups will go through each bag and see how many items were placed in the same bags. The leader will ask the participants to collectively decide what items belong in certain categories. If there is more than one answer decided on, their reasoning will have to be explained.

Last, the group will sit in a circle and look through the brochures and pamphlets and discuss the opportunities available at various community agencies. The group will then collectively decide which agency to attend as the group's community out-trip.

**Debriefing Questions/Closure:**

1. Look through all the information in the bags and pick at least three agencies that interest you most. Out of those three, which one do you want to go to the most? Why does that one agency interest you the most?

2. Once an agency has been picked for a field trip, how will you go about arranging the details of the trip?

3. If anything, what will you need to bring along with you on the trip?

**Leadership Considerations:**

1. The leader should be sure to obtain a wide variety of resources, but not so many that it gets confusing.

2. The leader should be sure to let the participants choose where their trip will take place—it is their trip.

**Variation:**

Instead of using community resources, the leader may use resources participants can utilize at home.

**Creator:** Amy Conron, Illinois State University, Normal, Illinois.

# Decisions, Decisions

**Space Requirements:** Classroom or activity room

**Equipment/Resource Requirements:** Pens or pencils, accompanying form

**Group Size:** Small group

**Program Goals:**
1. To increase participants' ability to make positive decisions.
2. To increase participants' ability to distinguish between positive and negative choices and decisions.

**Program Description:**
**Preparation:**
The leader will make copies of the Decisions, Decisions work sheet and/or alter the content of the work sheet as needed. The leader will place the work sheets on a table and make sure there is one writing utensil and work sheet for each participant.

**Introduction:**
The purposes of this activity are to assist participants in decision making and distinguishing between positive and negative decisions.

It is suggested that the leader begin the session with a discussion on the process of decision making. An example of a discussion is as follows:

Everyone makes decisions every day of their lives. Can anyone give me an example of a decision they have had to make just recently? How did it feel to make that decision? Today we are going to do an activity that focuses on decisions. We will discuss the process of decision making as a group once we complete a related work sheet.

**Activity Description:**
The leader will ask all the participants to sit around the table and take a work sheet from the table. The leader then will ask that each participant follow along on the work sheet as the leader reads the content of the work sheet aloud.

Once the work sheet has been read aloud, the leader will ask participants to write down a possible solution to the decision or what they would do if the decision was theirs to make. The participants should be given approximately five minutes to reply to each of the situations on the work sheet.

Once all of the participants are done writing answers, the leader will ask the participants to take turns discussing their answers. To begin, the leader may choose to answer one as an opener.

After all situations have been discussed, the leader should summarize the intent of the activity goals. The leader should use the debriefing questions to promote discussion.

**Debriefing Questions/Closure:**
1. How did you reach your decisions for each of the scenarios?
2. Would you consider your decision a positive choice or a negative choice?
3. How could you create a more positive choice?
4. How important are the daily decisions that we make?
5. What is a recent decision you made and what were the consequences?
6. Name some ways to tell if the decisions you are making are positive ones.
7. How does it feel to make a positive choice?

**Leadership Considerations:**
1. The leader should be familiar with the cognitive abilities of the participants.
2. The leader should not force participants to share their answers.

3. The leader should create a nonthreatening environment.

**Variations:**

1. The leader may modify the work sheet so that its content is applicable to both the agency (or program) and where the participants live.

2. The leader may divide the group into two teams and have them role-play the scenario and the decision they would make while in that particular situation.

3. If participants cannot read, the leader may discuss the scenarios and their answers verbally.

**Creator:** Amy Conron, Illinois State University, Normal, Illinois.

# Decisions, Decisions

1. You are playing ball in the park with your friends when a stranger approaches and asks if you would like to try some real fun. The stranger pulls out a bag filled with drugs and offers it to you and your group of friends. What would you do in this situation?

2. You have been invited to a roller skating party with your friends. You would like to go but you do not know how to skate and don't want to be embarrassed in front of your friends. What would you do in this situation?

3. You want to participate in a soccer league but your mother insists that you continue your piano lessons. The two are held at the same time. What could you do?

4. You have been receiving 50 cents a week for your allowance and you now want an increase. Your caretaker has already said that 50 cents a week is plenty for someone your age. What will you do to solve the problem?

# House of Cards

**Space Requirements:** Classroom or activity room

**Equipment/Resource Requirements:** Three decks of cards

**Group Size:** Small group

**Program Goals:**
1. To increase participants' ability to cooperate with peers.
2. To increase participants' ability to participate in group decisions.

**Program Description:**
**Preparation:**
The leader will obtain three decks of cards. If the group will be working on tables, the leader should make sure the tables are sturdy and do not wobble.

**Introduction:**
The leader will explain to the participants that they will be doing an activity that will require good cooperation and listening skills and good fine motor control.

**Activity Description:**
The leader will begin the activity by dividing participants into three equal groups. The leader will distribute one deck of cards to each group. Each group member gets an equal number of cards. Using the cards, the group members are to work together to build a one-level house. In turn, each group member will place one card in the house structure. (To begin, all members will need to place their cards simultaneously to build the walls.) The leader will explain that the cards are not to be creased or folded in any way. When this step is completed, the team should continue and build a two-level house out of cards.

After each level is completed, the team should continue until all cards have been used. The groups should do this task on their own, us-ing problem-solving, cooperation and teamwork skills to the level needed. After all teams have used all cards, the leader will go over the following questions.

**Debriefing Questions/Closure:**
1. What kind of skills had to be used to make this activity successful?
2. What kind of teamwork skills worked, what did not work too well?
3. Did someone in your group act as the leader? How did you determine who this person would be?
4. Was the contribution among group members about equal?
5. How were decisions made concerning where the cards would be placed?
6. What would you do differently next time?

**Leadership Considerations:**
1. The leader should have an example available of a multilevel house of cards, to demonstrate that it is possible to do.
2. The leader should make sure to keep the teams apart and place distance between the teams to prevent accidents.

**Variations:**
1. The leader may ask the participants to build different structures.
2. The participants may use other materials such as toothpicks and marshmallows.
3. The leader may establish different rules to reinforce different goals, e.g., establish that sets of partners need to determine where their cards go, each person build his or her own house.

**Creator:** Jennifer Matkowich, Illinois State University, Normal, Illinois.

# What If?

**Space Requirements:** Classroom or activity room

**Equipment/Resource Requirements:** Accompanying form, pens, pencils

**Group Size:** Small group

**Program Goals:**
1. To increase participants' awareness of decision making as a part of everyday life.
2. To increase participants' understanding of the consequences of decisions.

**Program Description:**
**Preparation:**
The leader needs to make enough copies of the What If? work sheet before starting the activity.

**Introduction:**
The purpose of this activity is to increase participants' awareness of the importance of decision making. The leader can begin the activity by initiating a discussion on making daily decisions.

**Activity Description:**
The leader will begin the activity with a description of decision making in everyday life and the consequences of making decisions. Next, the leader will distribute one work sheet to each participant and read each question aloud. The leader should ask the group members if they understand each question clearly. The participants should be given ample time to fill in answers.

To begin discussion, the leader may open by having completed a personal work sheet and sharing answers with the group. Next, the leader should encourage the participants to discuss their answers by randomly asking participants to share their answers.

The leader should focus on the outcomes and effects of different decisions made by different participants. The leader should emphasize that each decision an individual makes has consequences.

**Debriefing Questions/Closure:**
1. How did you make your decisions to answer the way you did?
2. How did your answers differ from everyone else's?
3. How do decisions we make affect us?
4. What's an example of a time when you could have made a more positive decision?
5. Why is thinking about the outcome or consequence important to consider before we make a decision?
6. How will you use what you've learned here today?

**Leadership Considerations:**
1. The leader should not demand participants share their answers if they appear reluctant.
2. The leader should emphasize and encourage participants to use positive answers.
3. The leader should allow enough time for the participants to explain their answers.

**Variations:**
1. Instead of using paper and pencil, the participants may state their answers and the leader may write some of the answers on a board. The group should discuss how different people make different decisions.
2. The leader may pose a "What If?" to the group and allow them to process it as a group.
3. The leader may allow the group to create "What If?" situations.

**Creator:** Amy Conron, Illinois State University, Normal, Illinois.

# What If?

1. If I won a million dollars, I would. . . .

2. If I could go to one place in the world, I would go to. . . .

3. If I could visit with one person I haven't seen in a long time, that person would be. . . .

4. If I could play one sport professionally for one day, that sport would be. . . .

5. If I met a famous person, I would want that person to be. . . .

6. If I could fly for one day, I would fly to. . . .

7. If I could say one nice thing to someone today, it would be. . . .

8. If I could eat any food I wanted, it would be. . . .

9. If I could do my favorite activity, it would be. . . .

10. If I could spend time with one person today, it would be. . . .

11. If I could learn one new leisure skill, it would be. . . .

12. If I could win one ticket to an event, the event would be. . . .

# Planning a Day Out

**Space Requirements:** Classroom or activity room

**Equipment/Resource Requirements:** Telephone books, paper, pencils, accompanying form

**Group Size:** Small group

**Program Goals:**
1. To increase participants' ability to make decisions about their leisure.
2. To increase participants' ability to accept responsibility for their own leisure decisions.
3. To increase participants' ability to compromise with peers.
4. To increase participants' ability to plan for leisure.

**Program Description:**

**Preparation:**

The leader will prepare work sheets and gather supplies. The leader may want to complete one work sheet as an example.

**Introduction:**

The purpose of the activity is to let participants work together in planning a day out and to demonstrate cooperation skills.

**Activity Description:**

The activity will open with a discussion about the importance of planning for leisure. Participants are given a phone book and a time schedule for one day. The schedule is divided into two-hour increments. The day begins at 10:00 A.M. and ends at 6:00 P.M. The group then is given instructions to plan the day with leisure activities of their choice. At this point it may be necessary for the leader to explain what leisure activities are. Also, the leader should explain to the group that it is important to plan the day well, because once an activity is written into a time slot, it may not be changed, except by agreement of the group.

Once all activities are chosen and all time slots are filled in, participants need to write down whatever they think may be needed to engage in the particular activity (i.e., equipment and money). This may include calling ahead for times, ticket prices, or reservations.

Each participant is allowed to decide on his or her own activities or work with a partner. However, in the end, all participants must work as a group to decide on which activities will be done in each time slot. If two or more different activities are planned for the same time slot, each participant should be able to give an explanation of why one particular activity should be chosen over another.

Once the planning is agreed on and completed, the entire group and the leader will work together to make the necessary arrangements to plan the day that has been decided upon. By knowing ahead of time that choosing an activity means that it must be carried out, participants will have to take responsibility for their decisions. Increasing skills such as assertiveness and activity planning will in turn be a good basis for leadership ability.

The leader should use the following debriefing questions to close this session and plan for the next.

**Debriefing Questions/Closure:**
1. What things did you find most difficult about this activity? What things did you find least difficult about this activity?
2. What has to be considered to make a decision about your leisure?
3. How well did the group members compromise about their decisions?
4. How satisfied are you with the planned day?
5. What did you learn about planning your leisure activities?
6. What do you need to do to get ready for the out-trip?

**Leadership Consideration:**
Depending on the background of the participants, the leader may give assistance to begin the activity regarding time scheduling.

**Variations:**
1. If the activity is too difficult for the participants, a list of different options for different time slots could be compiled by the leader ahead of time and given to the participants. The participants could use this list rather than a phone book to decrease the level of difficulty.
2. The leader may add in a limited monetary figure for the participants to work around.

**Creator:** Jessica Kamm, Illinois State University, Normal, Illinois.

# Planning a Day Out

## Your Day

**10 A.M.:** _____

_____

_____

_____

_____

_____

**12 Noon:** _____

_____

_____

_____

_____

_____

**2 P.M.:** _____

_____

_____

_____

_____

_____

**4 P.M.:** _____

_____

_____

_____

_____

_____

# What to Do?

**Space Requirements:** Classroom or activity room

**Equipment/Resource Requirements:** Accompanying questions, blank 3-by-5-inch cards

**Group Size:** Small group

**Program Goals:**
1. To increase participants' ability to make decisions.
2. To increase participants' ability to solve problems.

**Program Description:**
**Preparation:**
The leader should prepare the situation cards by typing the questions on 3-by-5-inch cards. The leader will place the cards in the middle of a table or floor and have the participants sit in a circle around the cards.

**Introduction:**
The purpose of this activity is to help participants use problem-solving and decision-making skills in various situations. The leader will explain the purpose and procedures to the group. The leader may say something like this:

> Has anyone ever been in a situation where there was a tough decision to be made? Would anyone like to give an example of a situation with a tough decision? Was it hard to make the decision? Today we are going to play a game that allows you to make decisions.

**Activity Description:**
Each participant will take a turn and pick one card from the pile. He or she will read the situation written on the card aloud and answer the question. The leader or group will decide if it is an *appropriate* answer. After each turn with an

appropriate answer, the other participants can have an opportunity to speak if they would have answered the question differently.

When the participant answers appropriately, he or she will get a point. Each participant wants to obtain a certain amount of points. The leader can decide the amount. A good number for a small group of participants is five.

When a participant does not answer appropriately, the question goes back into the pile. If the participant does answer appropriately the question should not go back into the pile.

The leader should offer help where needed. The leader should stress that there are no winners and losers; that everyone wants to try and get the maximum amount of points.

After taking time to discuss each situation fully, the leader will summarize the goals of the activity. The following debriefing questions can be used for closure.

**Debriefing Questions/Closure:**
1. Can anyone think of a situation where you've had to make a difficult decision?
2. How do you usually go about making a difficult decision?
3. Who influences you when you make decisions?
4. How do you know you're making a good decision? How do you know you're making a bad decision?
5. What are the end results or consequences of making a good decision? What are the end results or consequences of making a bad decision?
6. What makes a decision either a good one or a bad one?

**Leadership Considerations:**
1. The leader should know different additional problems to address to the group, making sure the content of the situations is at their level of understanding.

2. The leader should make sure to announce ahead of time the ways to receive points.
3. Participants can sit in a circle.

**Variations:**
1. New questions can be added to address a specific problem.

2. The leader may have the participants write their own situations on the cards.

**Creator:** Courtney Stauffer, Illinois State University, Normal, Illinois.

# What to Do?

## Situations for Playing Cards

- When you are playing outside, a bee stings you on the arm. The skin around the sting turns red and begins to swell. It hurts. What do you do?
- You are playing outside. All of a sudden, your left ankle twists and you fall down. Your ankle is throbbing with pain. What do you do?
- You are playing basketball with your friends. One accidentally hits you above your eye with his elbow. The area above your eye gets red and puffy. It then turns black and blue. What do you do?
- What would you do if while you were with two of your good friends, they start to get into a big argument?
- What would you tell your friend if he or she offered you a cigarette?
- What would you do if a stranger said, "Come here, I want to give you something?"
- How would you introduce yourself to someone new?
- What would you do if someone took your favorite book without asking?
- What do you do if a teacher asks you a question you don't know?
- What would you do if you accidentally did the wrong homework assignment? You didn't realize it was wrong until you were at school.
- While you are in class, you realize that you are confused about what you are supposed to do for homework. What do you do?
- What would you do if you went to the store with your friend and he started to shoplift?
- You have to buy some art supplies for school. When you get to the counter to pay you realize you didn't bring your money. What do you do?
- You are walking in the shopping center when you realize you don't know where you are? What do you do?
- While you are walking on the sidewalk, a stray dog comes by you. You do not know this dog. What do you do?
- While you are in school taking a test, the person sitting next to you asks you to give him an answer. What do you do?

- What would you do if there was another kid in your class and no one ever talked to him? They think he is stuck up, but he is just shy.
- What would you do if you had a headache and your friend offered you some of her prescription medicine?
- While you are walking down the street with your friend, you see a car running with no one in it. Your friend wants to hop in it and take it for a ride. What do you do?
- It is the night of the NBA basketball championship game. Your favorite team is playing and it starts in 20 minutes. You haven't even started on your homework that is due the next day. What do you do?
- You are in class with a substitute teacher. While she is facing the chalkboard, your friend throws his pencil at her. What would you do?
- What would you do if your friend in class was making fun of the quiet girl sitting next to you?
- While you are at a movie theater, a man behind you is slurping his soda so loudly that you can't hear the movie. What do you do?
- You are walking down the hall at school and you *accidentally* bump someone and his or her books fall on the floor. What do you do?
- You are with your friend in the gym, and he starts writing graffiti on the wall. What do you do?
- What would you do if you went into the bathroom and there were pills left on the counter?
- What would you do if the power went out while you were watching television at night?
- During the night, you wake up coughing. Your eyes burn. You smell smoke. Everyone else is still asleep. What do you do?
- While you are playing at the park with your friends, a stray dog wanders into the area. One of your friends runs over to pet the dog. What would you do?
- One afternoon, you are outside playing soccer. The sky grows dark. Rain begins to fall. You hear loud claps of thunder and see bolts of lightning. What do you do?

# To Agree or Disagree

**Space Requirements:** Classroom or activity room

**Equipment/Resource Requirements:** One sign that says Agree, one sign that says Disagree, masking tape, discussion list

**Group Size:** Small group

**Program Goals:**
1. To increase participants' awareness of people holding different opinions.
2. To increase participants' awareness of the importance of respecting others' opinions.
3. To improve participants' ability to resolve and appropriately react to conflict.
4. To increase participants' awareness of the effects of negatively reacting to conflict situations.

**Program Description:**
**Preparation:**
Prior to beginning the activity, the leader should tape the Agree sign on one side of the activity room and the Disagree sign on the opposite side of the room. He or she should also prepare a list of statements such as:

1. Being truthful is important, regardless of who it may hurt.
2. What's mine is mine, what's yours is mine.
3. You should respect others' privacy.
4. When two people disagree, they should compromise.
5. Stealing candy is okay, because it's just candy.
6. The best person always wins.
7. Fighting is a good solution when you disagree.
8. Making and keeping friends is important.
9. Friendships take time to build.
10. Listening to others is important.
11. Money buys happiness.
12. Leisure time should be used wisely.
13. Everyone has the potential to be a superstar.
14. How you treat others tells a lot about who you are.
15. You can only succeed by following the rules.

**Introduction:**
The leader should explain to the group members that they will be participating in an activity that will allow them to exercise decision-making skills and explain the opinions they hold and why they hold those opinions.

**Activity Description:**
The leader should explain to the group that he or she is going to read a variety of statements aloud. For example, the leader might say: "Conflicts should be settled peacefully." After each statement is read, each participant should walk to the Agree or Disagree sign that represents his or her opinion on that particular statement.

After participants walk to their area of designation, the leader will ask them to explain why they agree or disagree. The leader should encourage each person to be positive in stating why he or she agrees or disagrees and not to use any negative comments.

After calling out numerous statements, the leader will bring the group back together for discussion. The focus of the discussion should relate to explaining that not everyone thinks the same way or has the same opinions. As a result of this, conflicts may arise at some point in one's life. If and when this happens, it is important to be positive in resolving a conflict. Negative reactions should not be exercised, they will not help the situation. Also, the leader should emphasize that having a different opinion is not necessarily a bad thing. It is important for each person to be unique.

**Debriefing Questions/Closure:**

1. Has anyone here ever had to deal with a conflict that was the result of a difference of opinion? How did you deal with it?
2. How do you plan to exercise what you learned from participating in this activity?

**Leadership Considerations:**

1. The leader should make sure the statements are at the understanding level of the group.

2. The leader should make sure the group understands what opinions are and what conflicts are.

**Variations:**

1. The leader may focus on conflicts that often occur with siblings, friends, or parents.
2. The participants may role-play conflict resolution techniques.

**Creator:** Sandra Larson, Illinois State University, Normal, Illinois.

# Who Painted the Door?

**Space Requirements:** Classroom or activity room

**Equipment/Resource Requirements:** Playing cards made from accompanying information

**Group Size:** Small group

**Program Goals:**
1. To increase participants' small group cooperation skills.
2. To increase participants' ability to solve problems.

**Program Description:**

**Preparation:**
The leader will cut out the cards and divide them among the participants.

**Introduction:**
The purpose of the activity is to increase participants' group cooperation and problem-solving skills. The leader will explain the procedures to the participants.

The following is a suggestion for introducing the activity:

> Who likes to be a detective? Has anybody ever solved a mystery before? Today we are going to be detectives. We are trying to find who painted the door. There are many clues to the mystery and you, as a group, have to work together to solve it.

**Activity Description:**
The participants will work at a table, where they will all be able to easily see the cards. The leader will pass the cards out to each participant and explain the rules. Once the cards have been passed out, the group has to try to figure out who painted the door. Together they will have to find a way on their own to solve the mystery. The cards will be mixed up—some will be object cards, some will be place cards, some will be people cards, and the rest will be clue cards.

The leader will reinforce that they need to work together. The leader will offer assistance to the participants when needed. When they discover who painted the door, they will discuss with the leader how they found the painter. The leader will use the following questions for closure.

**Debriefing Questions/Closure:**
1. Has anyone ever solved a mystery?
2. How is a mystery like solving problems?
3. When you are solving a mystery with a group, how important is it to work well together?
4. If everyone tried to solve the problem by themselves, how far would the group get?
5. What kinds of problems do you try to solve every day?
6. How do other people help you solve problems?

**Leadership Considerations:**
1. The participants might need hints on how to start solving the mystery.
2. The leader should limit the group size to a maximum of five people, so the participants have more than one card.

**Variations:**
1. The leader may have the participants create their own mystery.
2. The leader may put different participants in charge of finding the painter, the supplies and the places.

**Creator:** Courtney Stauffer, Illinois State University, Normal, Illinois.

---

*Answer:* Tammy Tom Tom with the paint roller in the skyscraper.

# Who Painted the Door?

## Suspects

Phil Flip Flop

Adam Art

Mary Money

Tammy Tom Tom

Buster Bones

Ned North

## Supplies

Paintbrush

Paint Roller

Markers

Nail Polish

Spray Paint

Squirt Bottle

## Places

House

Apartment

Skyscraper

Store

Church

Car

## Clues

If the paintbrush was the weapon, then Buster Bones did it.

Phil Flip Flop is the only one to use markers.

The painted door was not at the apartment.

Tammy Tom Tom was at the skyscraper.

Tammy Tom Tom had a paint roller.

The squirt bottle was at the apartment.

Phil Flip Flop did not do it.

The spray paint was in the car.

Ned North had the only squirt bottle.

Phil Flip Flop was at the house.

It did not happen at the church.

The paintbrush was at the church.

Adam Art and Mary Money were in the car.

Only one person painted the door.

# Planning a Pizza Party!

**Space Requirements:** Classroom or activity room

**Equipment/Resource Requirements:** Telephone book, paper, writing utensils, local pizza coupon (if available), access to telephone

**Group Size:** Small group

**Program Goals:**
1. To increase participants' group cooperation and negotiation skills.
2. To increase participants' ability to plan for leisure events.
3. To increase participants' ability to make co-operative decisions.
4. To increase participants' ability to take responsibility for a decision.

**Program Description:**
**Preparation:**
The leader will have all the equipment spread around the table.

**Introduction:**
The purpose of the activity is to have the participants work together to plan a pizza party.

A suggestion for introducing the activity is as follows:

Has anyone ever planned a party before? What kind of party did you plan? Was it successful? Did anyone else help you plan? You as a group are going to be planning a pizza party. We will have the party at a later date, but you need to plan everything today. Keep in mind that you can either make or order the pizzas.

**Activity Description:**
The participants will sit around the table and plan for the party. They will need to plan what they need for the party including kind of pizza, how many pizzas, where the pizza will come from, whether they are ordering or making the pizzas, what toppings, what types of drinks, and how much money. The leader should try and allow the participants to figure out the answers to all of the these questions. If they are forgetting something or leaving something out, the leader should give them advice. The leader should encourage positive talking and that everyone needs to take a responsibility.

The leader will close the planning session with a summary of the decisions made and the date when the pizza will be made or ordered. The leader will debrief the group with the following questions.

**Debriefing Questions/Closure:**
1. How much did each of you contribute to the final decisions about the pizzas?
2. What kinds of compromise skills do you need for group decisions such as this?
3. What were the points of agreement?
4. What were the points of disagreement?
5. What are the benefits of everyone having a say in the final decisions?
6. What are the disadvantages of everyone having a say in the final decisions?
7. What did you learn from this activity?

**Leadership Considerations:**
1. The leader should allow one person to be in charge of making the phone calls for prices.
2. The leader should only offer help when the participants have forgotten things.

3. The leader should allow the participants to make their own compromises so they learn to compromise.
4. This is a great activity for the end of a session or program. It is a goal the participants can work toward.

**Variations:**
1. The participants may plan another type of party (ice cream, pasta, sixties).
2. The leader may have each participant plan a certain part of the party.

**Creator:** Courtney Stauffer, Illinois State University, Normal, Illinois.

# What Is a Consequence?

**Space Requirements:** May be done outdoors or indoors

**Equipment/Resource Requirements:** Plastic eggs, slips of paper with various situations (see examples)

**Group Size:** Small group

**Program Goals:**
1. To increase participants' knowledge of consequences they might encounter in certain situations.
2. To improve participants' decision-making skills.

**Program Description:**
**Preparation:**
The leader will place the provided situations on small slips of paper and place them inside the plastic eggs. The following situations go in the eggs:

1. I'm getting really mad at Charlie right now and am thinking about kicking him.
2. I think I'll skip doing my homework and watch TV all night instead.
3. I know that kid did bad on his test so I'm going to call him stupid.
4. The list of spelling words is so long—I think I'll just wait till tomorrow to copy it.
5. I know the teacher told us to listen carefully but I feel like talking right now.
6. The teacher told me to sit in this seat, but I want to sit on the other side of the room.
7. I want the game that Taneisha has in her hand.
8. I want a snack right now.
9. It's bedtime and I don't want to take a bath.
10. It's time to get up and I don't want to get out of bed.

11. If I do a sloppy job on my homework, I'm sure nobody will notice.
12. I'm going to call that overweight boy coming in the door "Fatty."
13. I want to play outside in the rain.
14. Richard wants to watch a video, and I want to watch television.
15. I don't want that stuff that stings on my scratched knee.
16. I want to spend all my money on candy.
17. I'm going to run away.
18. Certainly, shoplifting candy won't get me in trouble.

**Introduction:**
The leader will explain to the group that it is important for people to think through what might happen before they act on a situation. This activity will present the concept of consequences and provide situations to consider what might happen as a result of their actions. At this time, it may be necessary for the leader to explain these concepts by giving various examples.

**Activity Description:**
The leader will explain to the group members that they are going on an egg hunt. What will be found in the eggs may not be what they are used to finding. The rules of the hunt are as follows:

- Everyone will be allowed to pick up only one egg.
- If the participants spot more than one egg, they are not to tell the others the location of that egg. Each person should find his or her egg on his or her own.
- After getting an egg, the participants will return to the "Egg" area (location to be chosen by leader).
- The participants should not open and read the slip of the paper in their egg until instructed to do so by the leader.

Once everyone returns to the "Egg" area, the group will have a short discussion. The leader will instruct the group to form a circle. The leader will have each of the participants remove the slip of paper from his or her egg. Starting with the first person who returned to the "Egg" area, the leader will have the participants read their situations. Next, the leader will have them tell the group what might happen as a consequence if they didn't think through the situation. What might happen if they acted on these thoughts? The group will discuss each situation thoroughly. The leader will close the session with the following debriefing questions.

**Debriefing Questions/Closure:**
1. Explain that a consequence is something that happens because of something that you do. There can be good consequences and not so good consequences. What are some examples of each?
2. What are some situations that you have been in that resulted in positive consequences? What are some situations that you have been in that resulted in negative consequences?
3. Does every action or decision have some kind of consequence?
4. What do you have to do to not have negative consequences?

**Leadership Considerations:**
1. The leader will reinforce to the participants that they may only find one egg.
2. The leader will encourage the participants to listen to each other's situations and comments.

**Variations:**
1. This activity can be modified to discuss any topic.
2. If this is done indoors, the participants may enjoy finding the eggs in a dark room with a flashlight.

**Creator:** Amanda L. McGowen, Illinois State University, Normal, Illinois.

# Growing Grounds

**Space Requirements:** Classroom or activity room

**Equipment/Resource Requirements:** Seeds (such as corn, barley, alfalfa, lentils, soybeans, rye, peas, lima beans, or sunflower), widemouthed quart jar, bulb pan or clay saucer, water, potting soil, pots, sprouting tray

**Group Size:** Small group

**Program Goals:**
1. To increase participants' feelings of responsibility.
2. To improve participants' feelings of self-worth and accomplishment.

**Program Description:**
**Preparation:**
The leader will have seeds (separated by types), quart jar of water, and sprouting tray available for participants.

**Introduction:**
The purpose of this activity is to introduce participants to a project that is fun and places an emphasis on personal responsibility through an ongoing project rather than a one-day completed product.

**Activity Description:**
The participants will soak the seeds in water for 24 hours. After 24 hours, they should drain the seeds and place them into the quart jar in a warm, dark environment. Participants are to rinse and drain the seeds one to two times daily. (Within two weeks the seeds will sprout.) The participants should plant their seeds in the pots with the potting soil (seeds should be planted about an inch below the surface). Within two to fourteen days, the plants will emerge.

Each time the participant rinses the seeds, the leader and group will talk about responsibility for living things. The leader will discuss taking care of plants as a leisure option. When the plants are fully growing, the leader will gather the group to discuss the debriefing questions.

**Debriefing Questions/Closure:**
1. What were your responsibilities for this project?
2. What would have happened if you did not follow through with your responsibilities of the activity on a daily basis?
3. What are some everyday responsibilities you have?
4. How does it make you feel to be responsible for something?
5. What happens when you don't follow through with your responsibilities?
6. Why is it important to be responsible?
7. What happens when you make the decision to not be responsible?

**Leadership Considerations:**
1. The leader should give suggestions on what to do with the plants after they are fully grown.
2. The leader should give suggestions on how to further acquire responsibilities in everyday life.

**Variations:**
1. The leader may make the activity an at-home activity. The leader may have the participants be solely responsible for the seedlings and their growth.
2. The leader may include an informational section about where the seeds originated or what uses they have had in the past.

3. The leader may choose to use other types of seeds, such as flower seeds.
4. The leader may ask a gardener or horticulturist to bring plants and discuss their growth with the children.

5. The leader may create a follow-up activity that will use the plants.

**Creator:** Kristen Boys, Illinois State University, Normal, Illinois.

# What Barrier?

**Space Requirements:** Classroom or activity room

**Equipment/Resource Requirements:** Accompanying forms, chalkboard, pencils or pens, bag or hat, playing cards, tape

**Group Size:** Small group

**Program Goals:**
1. To improve participants' ability to identify potential barriers to a satisfying leisure lifestyle.
2. To improve participants' ability to make appropriate decisions to overcome barriers related to leisure participation.

**Program Description:**
**Preparation:**
*Note:* This activity was designed primarily for individuals with substance abuse problems.

The leader will make the appropriate number of copies of the accompanying form and arrange the room—participants will be divided into four groups. The leader will attach one playing card to the bottom of each chair—allow only the number of chairs as are participants.

**Introduction:**
The purpose of this activity is to help participants identify barriers to leisure and ways to eliminate or reduce them.

**Activity Description:**
The leader should begin by stating the purpose and goals of this activity. The leader will have participants brainstorm possible barriers to leisure. Possible barriers include:

- cannot find a baby-sitter;
- cannot participate without chemical or substance abuse;
- facilities overcrowded;
- family commitment;
- fear of the unknown;
- inability to identify or use personal resources for leisure involvement;
- inability to take responsibility for leisure involvement;
- inadequate knowledge of what equipment or materials to use;
- inadequate knowledge of where to go to do activity;
- inadequate planning and decision-making skills;
- inadequate social skills;
- lack of experience—no confidence to explore new areas of leisure;
- lack of making leisure a priority;
- lack of money;
- lack of opportunity to participate near home;
- lack of skills;
- lack of time;
- lack of transportation;
- no or little appreciation for leisure;
- not accepted because of gender (social/cultural);
- not physically able to participate;
- partner or friend not interested in trying a new activity;
- preconceived notions of what leisure should be;
- problems finding leisure partners; and
- weather.

The leader will write ideas on the chalkboard. The leader will determine which barriers are real and which are perceived.

Next, the participants will reach under their chair and detach the playing card. They will split into groups based on the suit of their playing card.

The leader will pass out the pencils and pens and have each group pull three scenarios from the hat. Each group will also be given the scenario about participation without chemical or substance abuse (groups should have a total of four scenarios).

The participants will brainstorm (in groups) possible ways to overcome the barriers presented. The participants should be given 10–15 minutes to brainstorm.

Before discussion, the leader will hand out the scenario sheet (intact) to each participant. The leader will instruct the participants to write down the ideas generated by the upcoming discussion.

Each group will read its barrier scenarios along with the ideas generated to overcome barriers. The leader will encourage discussion between groups (i.e., Do these ideas seem realistic? Can anyone add additional suggestions? Has anyone tried this idea to overcome the barrier?). All groups will share ideas for the chemical or substance abuse scenario after each group has shared all other scenarios.

The leader will review the purpose and goals of the activity. The leader will restate the goals and use the following debriefing questions.

**Debriefing Questions/Closure:**
1. As a result of this activity, will you feel more confident in dealing with potential barriers to leisure after treatment?
2. What scenarios would you add to this activity?
3. What barrier is most troublesome to your leisure?
4. What ways have you learned to overcome barriers?
5. What will you do the next time you encounter a barrier?

**Leadership Considerations:**
1. The leader should be familiar with leisure barriers and ideas for overcoming barriers.
2. The leader should encourage participants to come up with realistic suggestions.

**Variations:**
1. When using the activity for individuals or small groups, the leader may have the participant(s) work individually on one barrier scenario at a time and discuss after each.
2. For different participant populations and/or ages, the leader may change the scenarios to match common barriers for that group.

**Creator:** Susan Osborn, Illinois State University, Normal, Illinois.

# What Barrier?

## Overcoming Potential Barriers to Leisure

I do not have the skills necessary to participate in rock climbing.

1.

2.

3.

4.

I do not know where to find information about a local hiking club or if one even exists.

1.

2.

3.

4.

I am not sure what equipment is necessary for scuba diving.

1.

2.

3.

4.

I do not have time for the leisure activities I really want to do.

1.

2.

3.

4.

Leisure is just not important to me.

1.

2.

3.

4.

I am not very creative and do not think I would enjoy doing arts and crafts activities.

1.

2.

3.

4.

I love to swim, but every time I go to the public pool, it is so crowded I can't enjoy myself.

1.

2.

3.

4.

I want to try a new activity but my best friend will not try it with me (unfortunately, for this new activity I need a partner).

1.

2.

3.

4.

I just don't have the time for leisure activities.

1.

2.

3.

4.

I do not have the transportation to take advantage of many leisure activities I would like to do.

1.

2.

3.

4.

Every time I want to do something outside the weather is bad, so I just watch TV instead.

1.

2.

3.

4.

I am just physically not strong enough to participate in many active recreation activities.

1.

2.

3.

4.

I would like to learn a new activity that may be considered too masculine or feminine and I think my friends will laugh at me.

1.

2.

3.

4.

I can't go. The baby-sitter backed out or I could not find a baby-sitter.

1.

2.

3.

4.

I really try to do new things, it's everybody else who doesn't want to do anything.

1.

2.

3.

4.

I cannot participate without using alcohol or drugs.

1.

2.

3.

4.

# Recreation Roadblock Game

**Space Requirements:** Classroom or activity room

**Equipment/Resource Requirements:** Game board, cards, die, playing pieces

**Group Size:** Small group

**Program Goals:**
1. To increase participants' ability to identify potential barriers to a satisfying leisure lifestyle.
2. To increase participants' ability to make appropriate decisions to overcome barriers related to leisure participation.

**Program Description:**
**Preparation:**
The leader will create a game board on a large piece of cardboard (see rules for instructions) and gather all other supplies.

**Introduction:**
The purpose of this activity is to help participants identify potential barriers to leisure and ways to overcome those barriers.

**Activity Description:**
The leader begins by stating the purpose and goals of the activity. The leader and the group will discuss leisure barriers. The leader will ask the participants to state some leisure barriers that may be a problem for them currently. The leader will ask participants how they may be able to overcome those barriers.

The leader will introduce game and go over all rules (see accompanying game rules). The participants will play the game. As the game is going on, discussion will be inevitable. (Participants must match barrier cards with removal cards and the leader is final judge.)

The following are suggested processing questions (may be asked during and after game play):

1. Which Recreation Roadblock cards represent real barriers to leisure for you?
2. Which Roadblock Removal cards have you used to overcome a barrier to leisure?
3. Which Roadblock Removal card suggestions are feasible for you?
4. What additional leisure barriers do you face in your life?

The leader will close the activity by refocusing on the purpose and goals.

**Debriefing Questions/Closure:**
1. Name two barriers to your leisure.
2. Name two ways to overcome these barriers.
3. How will you use this information in the future?

**Leadership Considerations:**
1. The leader should be familiar with the game.
2. The leader should notice how players react to the barrier and removal cards and seize the opportunity to discuss how they personally feel about the barrier or the suggestion to overcome the barrier.
3. The participants may try to make matches that are inappropriate. When making a decision about a match, if the leader disagrees with the participant, the leader should explain his or her decision.

**Variations:**
1. All players finish and the player with the lowest number of Recreation Roadblock cards wins.
2. The leader may choose to discuss each "roadblock" (barrier) as the card is drawn.
3. The leader may use larger and/or heavier pieces for those individuals with low-level fine motor functioning.

4. The participants may play the game by using just the Roadblock Removal cards or just the Recreation Roadblock cards. The leader may have the participants guess what barrier it will help to overcome or how they can overcome the barrier.

5. The leader may make additional cards and add barriers that are common to the population he or she is working with.

**Creator:** Susan Osborn, Illinois State University, Normal, Illinois.

# Recreation Roadblock Game

## Rules of Play

**Object of Game:** To get rid of as many Recreation Roadblock cards as possible by making an appropriate match to a Roadblock Removal card and doing so before reaching the "finish" square.

**Playing the Game:**

1. Each player selects one Roadblock Removal card and one Recreation Roadblock card from the top of each pile. (*Note:* It is not necessary to keep cards a secret from other players, but a player may choose to do so.)
2. Each player rolls the die to determine who will start. The highest roll will begin the game.
3. The first player rolls the die and moves the number of spaces represented by the number on the die.
4. Upon arriving at the new playing square, the player follows the directions indicated (see Playing Cards and Game Board Squares instructions).
5. When a Recreation Roadblock card is matched with an appropriate Roadblock Removal card both cards are placed at the bottom of their piles. (For instance, if a player picks up a Recreation Roadblock card that states, "Lack of money" there are several cards that may work to get rid of this barrier—"Do similar activity that is less expensive" or "Budget for leisure and recreation activities." Either card will work.)
6. Making a match and returning roadblock and removal cards may be done at any time during the player's turn.
7. When the player makes a match, another turn is taken.

**Playing Cards:**

1. Recreation Roadblock Cards: These cards have leisure and recreation barriers printed on them. The player must find a Roadblock Removal card that matches.

2. Roadblock Removal Cards: These cards have a suggestion to overcome various barriers to leisure and recreation. The player must find a Recreation Roadblock card that matches.
3. Wild Cards: These cards are found in the Roadblock Removal card pile. The player is permitted to come up with a unique idea to overcome a barrier card he or she may hold. An automatic match is made.

**Game Board Squares:**

1. Yellow Squares: The yellow squares represent a Roadblock Removal card. Each time a player lands on one of the yellow squares, he or she must pick up a Roadblock Removal card.
2. Orange Squares: The orange squares represent a Recreation Roadblock card. Each time a player lands on one of the orange squares, he or she must pick up a Recreation Roadblock card.
3. Reading Squares: Each time a player lands on one of the reading squares, he or she must follow the instructions on the reading square:

   - Roll Again—Take another turn.
   - Move Forward—Move playing piece forward the number of spaces indicated.
   - Move Back—Move playing piece backward the number of spaces indicated.
   - Give a Recreation Roadblock Card to Player on Left/Right—The player turns his or her Roadblock cards facedown, shuffles and picks one to give to the player on his or her left or right.
   - Give a Roadblock Removal Card to Player on Left/Right—The player turns his or her Removal cards facedown, shuffles and picks one to give to the player on his or her left or right.
   - Take a Roadblock Removal Card from Player on Left/Right—The player picks

a Roadblock card from the player to the left or right (cards should be facedown).

- Take a Roadblock Removal Card from Player on Left/Right—The player picks a Removal card from the player to his or her left or right (cards should be facedown).

**Winning the Game:**

The first player to reach the "finish" square wins. An exact roll is not needed to win.

**Variations/Modifications:**

1. All players finish and player with the lowest number of Recreation Roadblock cards wins.
2. Although there are no time limitations with the original game, a time could be set and the winner is the player with lowest number of Recreation Roadblock cards when the time limit is reached.
3. Discuss each Roadblock (barrier) as the card is drawn.
4. Add Braille stickers to the board and cards.
5. Use larger and/or heavier pieces for those individuals with low-level fine motor functioning.
6. Additional blank cards can be included to add barriers specific to population.
7. Play the game by using just the Recreation Removal cards. Have players guess what barrier it will help to overcome.

**Suggested Discussion Questions:**

1. Which Roadblock cards represent real barriers to leisure or recreation for you?

2. Which Roadblock Removal cards have you used to overcome a barrier to leisure or recreation?
3. Which Roadblock Removal card suggestions are feasible to you? Which are not?
4. Which Roadblock Removal card suggestions will you try to incorporate into your life in order to participate in leisure and recreation activities?
5. What additional leisure barriers do you face in your life?
6. Has this game made you more aware of your own personal leisure and recreation barriers and how to overcome these barriers? How?

**Suggestions for Facilitating the Game:**

1. Before play begins, discuss leisure and recreation barriers. See if participants can come up with a few barriers. Ask participants how they can overcome the barriers mentioned.
2. Read rules aloud. Allow participants to ask clarification questions.
3. Each Recreation Roadblock card may have several appropriate Roadblock Removal cards. The leader will make the final decision to determine if the removal card is a solution to the roadblock (barrier). This also applies to the Wild Cards. The suggestions made must be realistic and appropriate. Do not make a decision without explaining your decision to the players.
4. Notice how players react to the Recreation Roadblock and Roadblock Removal cards. Seize the opportunity to discuss how they personally feel about the barrier or the suggestion to overcome the barrier.

# Puzzling

**Space Requirements:** Classroom or activity room

**Equipment/Resource Requirements:** Plastic bags, jigsaw puzzles with a riddle on the back (one puzzle for every two participants)

**Group Size:** Small group

**Program Goals:**
1. To increase participants' ability to problem solve with a partner.
2. To increase participants' verbalization of thought with a partner.

**Program Description:**
**Preparation:**
The leader should purchase or make one mini jigsaw puzzle for every two participants. The leader will write a riddle on the back of each puzzle.

**Introduction:**
The purpose of this activity is to improve participants' ability to solve problems and verbalize their thought processes with a partner.

**Activity Description:**
The leader will begin by stating the goals and purpose of the activity. The leader will ask participants to discuss some examples where they have problem solved to a good solution. The leader will have the mini puzzles separated into two bags per puzzle. The leader will pass out the bags to the group members as they arrive.

When the leader gives the command, the participants must find the person who has the matching puzzle pieces. They will put the puzzle together. Once the puzzle is put together, the participants will turn the puzzle over and solve the riddle on the back.

The first pair to complete the riddle, raise their hands, and tell the leader will win a prize.

The leader will close the activity by discussing the following debriefing questions.

**Debriefing Questions/Closure:**
1. How did you, as a pair, solve the puzzle?
2. What problems did you encounter while participating in this activity?
3. How did you handle or solve these problems?
4. What decisions did you have to make while participating in this activity?
5. What are some decisions you have to make every day?
6. What steps do you take to solve these problems or make these decisions?

**Leadership Considerations:**
1. The leader will tell the participants to cooperate with each other and work together.
2. The participants should try to work without help from the leader.
3. If participants need help, the leader should provide the same type and amount of assistance to each group.

**Variations:**
1. This activity could be used as an icebreaker to have participants get into groups or teams.
2. The activity could be made easier by already having pairs or teams and seeing which group puts the puzzle together and answers the riddle the fastest.

**Creator:** Renee Raczkowski, Illinois State University, Normal, Illinois.

# Leisure Awareness and Leisure Resources

# Where Is Leisure?

**Space Requirements:** Classroom or activity room

**Equipment/Resource Requirements:** Cutouts of leisure resources (from magazines), glue, construction paper, scissors

**Group Size:** Small group

**Program Goals:**
1. To increase participants' awareness of community and home leisure resources.
2. To increase participants' ability to exercise decision-making skills.
3. To increase participants' ability to follow directions and stay on task.

**Program Description:**
**Preparation:**
Prior to the activity, the leader should cut out a variety of leisure resource pictures (any thing or facility that can be used for leisure, such as fitness center, bicycle, computer, or park) from magazines. A completed example should be prepared to share with the group.

**Introduction:**
The purpose of this activity is to increase participants' awareness of home and community leisure resources, their ability to make decisions, and their ability to listen to and follow directions.

**Activity Description:**
The leader will begin by explaining that a leisure resource is any thing or any facility that can be used for leisure. Participants can be asked to give a few examples. The leader continues by holding up various pictures and asking the group if the picture represents a community or a home leisure resource. The group members will decide and the leader will tell them if their response is right or wrong. Answers may go both ways de-

pending on the actual resource. The leader then will put all pictures into one pile.

The group will be responsible for separating the pictures into two piles: community resources and home resources. After the pile has been separated, the leader will distribute one sheet of construction paper to each participant. The participants will be instructed to draw a line down the center of their paper. Next, they will write the title *Community* on one side and *Home* on the other. When this step is done, the participants will choose the leisure resources that are actually located in their community and home. They should glue these pictures onto their sheet under the correct heading. The leader will conclude the activity by discussing the following questions.

**Debriefing Questions/Closure:**
1. Have you used all of the leisure resources that you included in your picture?
2. What is your favorite leisure resource to use inside? What is your favorite leisure resource to use outside?
3. Who do you usually do these activities with?
4. What did you learn about things or places available for leisure in your community?
5. What did you learn about things available for leisure in your home?
6. When are good times to use these things?

**Leadership Considerations:**
1. It may be necessary to have a longer discussion about leisure resources before doing the activity, depending on the participants.
2. The leader should make sure the participants are putting resources under the correct headings.
3. The leader should encourage the participants to glue on only those resources they have used.

**Variations:**
1. The participants could draw leisure resources themselves.
2. The participants could look through magazines and cut out their own activities.

**Creator:** Connie Campbell, Illinois State University, Normal, Illinois.

# Pictures Say a Lot

**Space Requirements:** Classroom or activity room

**Equipment/Resource Requirements:** Accompanying work sheet, glue, magazines, markers or crayons

**Group Size:** Small group

**Program Goals:**
1. To increase participants' awareness of leisure resources located within the home environment.
2. To increase participants' ability to follow directions and remain on task.

**Program Description:**
**Preparation:**
The leader should gather all materials and set up the activity room. A completed example should be prepared to share with the group.

**Introduction:**
The leader will explain to the participants that they will be doing an activity that will focus on leisure resources located within their home environment. At this time it may be necessary for the leader to discuss what leisure resources are and provide examples.

**Activity Description:**
The leader will distribute a work sheet to each participant. The work sheet will have the frame of a house drawn on it. The other area on the work sheet represents the yard.

The leader will explain to participants that they need to draw a picture of themselves somewhere on the work sheet, either inside or outside of the house. The picture can be of just their face or a view of their whole body.

After doing this, the participants should look through the magazines and cut out pictures of leisure resources that they have located in their home environment. The resources must be those that they already own, and they can be resources located within or outside of the home. They then should paste the pictures in the appropriate location of their home. If they are unable to find a picture of a particular resource they can draw the resource with the markers and crayons.

The leader should give the participants 30–45 minutes to complete the activity. The leader will conclude by having each participant share his or her picture with the group and explain the leisure resources that he or she included. The group should discuss the following questions.

**Debriefing Questions/Closure:**
1. What is your favorite leisure resource to use inside?
2. What is your favorite leisure resource to use outside?
3. Who do you usually use these leisure resources with?
4. If you could do anything you want on a sunny Saturday morning, what would you do?
5. What additional leisure resources would you like to include on your picture?

**Leadership Considerations:**
1. The leader should instruct the participants to glue only on one side of the paper.
2. The leader should instruct the participants to choose only leisure resources and activities that are positive and healthy.
3. The leader should have a variety of magazines available, preferably age-appropriate.

**Variation:**
The leader may choose to use a larger piece of paper and have the participants include leisure resources available in their community.

**Creator:** Connie Campbell, Illinois State University, Normal, Illinois.

# Pictures Say a Lot

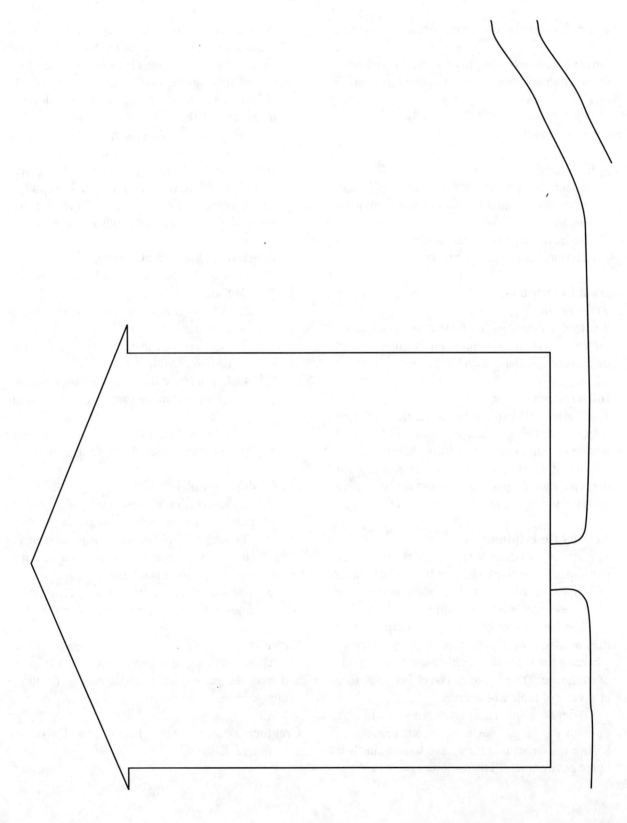

# Planting Your Own Garden

**Space Requirements:** Classroom or activity room

**Equipment/Resource Requirements:** Flower pots, potting soil, scoop for the soil, assorted seeds, newspapers

**Group Size:** Small group

**Program Goals:**
1. To increase participants' knowledge of gardening.
2. To increase participants' knowledge of alternative leisure activities.
3. To increase participants' sense of responsibility.

**Program Description:**

**Preparation:**
The leader should gather all the necessary supplies. Prior to beginning the activity the leader should lay down the newspapers on the work surface. One flowerpot should be placed in front of each participant. The soil and seeds should be in the middle of the working area, as these materials will be shared.

**Introduction:**
The purpose of this activity is to increase the participants' knowledge of gardening and alternative leisure activities. The leader should begin the activity with a discussion on what it takes to have a successful and healthy garden.

A suggestion for beginning the activity is as follows:

Gardening can be fun and exciting! Growing plants can be a very fulfilling task. However, for plants to grow successfully they need to be taken care of. Can anyone tell me some of the steps it takes to grow a garden? (Let the participants give their answers). Today we are going to build our own garden and watch it grow!

**Activity Description:**
The leader will begin the activity by asking the participants to pass around the bag of soil so that each individual can scoop out soil to fill his or her flowerpot. The pot should be filled to approximately one inch from the top.

Once the participants have filled their flowerpot with soil, the leader will ask them to take their fingers and make five holes in the soil approximately one-inch deep.

Next, the participants will take five seeds of their choice, plant them in the holes, and then cover the holes with soil. The participants then will add water to the pots and place them in an area that receives sunlight.

The leader will refocus on the goals of the activity and use the following debriefing questions to summarize the activity.

**Debriefing Questions/Closure:**
1. How will you take care of your seeds over the next few weeks?
2. What can you do with your plant when it becomes too big for its pot?
3. What did you learn about having your own garden?
4. Living things need to be taken care of. What responsibilities do you have to take care of these seeds?
5. How might you take care of plants as a hobby?

**Leadership Considerations:**
1. The leader should assist the participants if they appear to have difficulty filling their pot with soil.
2. The leader should watch attentively to ensure the participants handle the soil properly and do not misuse it.

3. The leader should instruct participants of the schedule they will have to maintain to continue to care for their plants.

**Variations:**

1. The group, as a whole, may plant one large garden in a large pot or outside, making it more of a cooperative activity.

2. The participants may plant a specific garden, such as a vegetable garden or a flower garden.

**Creator:** Amy Conron, Illinois State University, Normal, Illinois.

# Leisure Memory

**Space Requirements:** Classroom or activity room

**Equipment/Resource Requirements:** Index cards with words or phrases about leisure activities (two of each activity)

**Group Size:** Small group

**Program Goals:**
1. To increase participants' awareness of leisure activities.
2. To increase participants' short-term memory recall skills.

**Program Description:**
**Preparation:**
The leader should have all the cards prepared before the activity begins. Some examples of leisure and recreation cards are water skiing, sledding, swimming, volleyball, basketball, soccer, football, gardening, jumping rope, hiking, and going to an amusement park.

A variety of traditional and nontraditional activities are recommended. Two cards for each word or phrase should be created and all the cards should be shuffled well.

**Introduction:**
The purpose of this activity is to increase the participants' awareness of different types of leisure activities and increase the participants' ability to recall the placement of cards. The leader will explain the purpose and goals at the beginning of the activity and have the participants spread all the cards facedown on a flat surface such as the floor or table. The leader may begin the activity by asking the participants if they have ever played a memory game before.

**Activity Description:**
Once all the cards are spread out facedown on a flat surface, the leader will select who will go first. Play then will continue in a clockwise direction.

The first participant will flip over two cards. If the two cards match, the player takes the pair and is allowed to take another turn. If the cards do not match, the player needs to make sure all the other participants see the two cards before flipping them back over. The turn then goes to the next player and the same routine is followed.

Once all the cards have been matched correctly, the players count their doubles and the one with the most pairs is the winner.

The leader should close the activity by beginning a discussion about all the activities. The leader should have the participants pick some of the activities they enjoy and talk about them.

**Debriefing Questions/Closure:**
1. Was it difficult to remember where particular cards were after people flipped them over?
2. In which of the activities mentioned have you participated?
3. In which would you like to participate?
4. Where would you go to learn these activities?
5. Where would you go to participate in these activities?

**Leadership Considerations:**
1. The leader should make sure the participants are taking their correct turn and are waiting for the previous player to flip the cards back over.
2. The leader should create as many cards as possible to allow for variety and make the game more challenging.
3. The leader should assist the participants if they are having a difficult time reading what is on the card.

**Variations:**
1. One card could have a word on it and another a phrase. The players then match the word with the correct phrase.

2. The cards could be made with pictures instead of words or phrases.
3. An alternative category of cards could be used, i.e., hygiene, manners, school subjects.
4. The leader could make it a team memory game by dividing the participants into two groups.

5. The leader could have the group make the cards for one session and then play the game the next session.

**Creator:** Amy Conron, Illinois State University, Normal, Illinois.

# Messages About My Leisure Skills

**Space Requirements:** Classroom or activity room

**Equipment/Resource Requirements:** One large piece of drawing paper for each participant, markers, crayons, pencils, construction paper, glue and scissors

**Group Size:** Small group

**Program Goals:**
1. To increase participants' awareness of leisure skills.
2. To increase participants' awareness of their own personal leisure skills.

**Program Description:**
**Preparation:**
Prior to the activity, the leader will gather all of the necessary supplies and precut sheets of drawing paper (the paper needs to be large enough to trace a person's body on it). The leader may want to have an example prepared to use as a visual aid and to help promote discussion.

**Introduction:**
The main purpose of this activity is to increase participants' awareness of leisure skills that pertain to themselves. The leader can begin the activity by initiating a discussion about what types of activities each of the participants like to do or would like to do. The leader also can use his or her example to demonstrate to the participants what they need to do.

**Activity Description:**
The leader will divide the group into pairs. One participant will lie down on the paper while the other traces around the body. Once both partners have their bodies outlined, each will take his or her own outline.

On the outline of their body, the participants are asked to write what leisure skill they feel they are good at, enjoy or would like to participate in.

The participants need to write this on the body part that is required to do the activity. More than one body part may be necessary so they can write it several times. Participants can decorate their outline any way they would like.

Once they have completed drawing on their outline, they will be asked to share what they have written and drawn on their outline with the group and state why they chose the certain activities they did.

**Debriefing Questions/Closure:**
1. What types of leisure activity skills do you feel you are good at, enjoy or would like to learn?
2. What skills do you feel you need to improve upon?
3. Was it difficult to place certain activities on your outline?
4. What are the differences among each of the participants' interests? What are the similarities?
5. What are some of the activities you would like to do in the future? How can you go about getting involved in these?

**Leadership Considerations:**
1. The leader should pair up people who get along well or pair up two who don't normally work together.
2. The leader should use a creative system when pairing up people.
3. The leader should make sure back-up supplies are available.
4. The leader should be aware of some participants' privacy issues.

**Variations:**
1. Instead of identifying leisure skills, the participants could write down areas of strength.
2. After the participants have their body outlined, the leader may have all of the other participants write two positive things about each person on their outline.

3. Following the activity, the participants could hang the completed drawings on a bulletin board to display.

**Creator:** Amy Conron, Illinois State University, Normal, Illinois.

# Sports Memory

**Space Requirements:** Classroom or activity room

**Equipment/Resource Requirements:** Game index cards

**Group Size:** Small group

**Program Goals:**
1. To improve participants' awareness of sports.
2. To increase participants' short-term memory recall skills.

**Program Description:**
**Preparation:**
The leader should prepare index cards ahead of time. This process requires writing a variety of sports equipment on index cards. Examples of sports equipment include:

- baseball glove,
- baseball bat,
- basketball,
- basketball hoop,
- bridge cards,
- canoeing oar,
- fishing hook,
- fishing rod,
- football,
- golf ball,
- golf club,
- hockey puck,
- hockey stick,
- soccer ball, and
- tennis ball.

Each piece of sports equipment should be written on two index cards (as a pair). Also, each piece of sports equipment used should be age-appropriate. The total pairs of cards should equal approximately 20–25.

**Introduction:**
The leader should begin by explaining to the group members that they will be participating in a game that will challenge their short-term memory recall skills. It also will require them to exercise good concentration skills. In addition, from participating in this activity, they will have the opportunity to learn about new sports and sports equipment.

**Activity Description:**
The leader will spread the cards on a large table, facedown. The leader will explain to the participants that they will be taking turns turning the cards over. Each card has the name of a piece of sports equipment written on it. Each participant will be given the opportunity to turn two cards over. The object of the game is to try and find matches, e.g., two cards that say basketball.

Each participant should completely turn the card over so that each person in the group is able to see what is written on the card. If a match is made, that person should continue to turn over two cards at a time. If a match is not made, the cards should be turned facedown in their place.

As cards are viewed, the group can discuss the sport. Questions may be asked such as:

- Where would this sport be played?
- What equipment is needed to play this sport?
- How many people can play at one time?

The leader should close by refocusing on the goals and using the following questions.

**Debriefing Questions/Closure:**
1. To what new sports did this game introduce you?
2. In which of these sports have you participated? And in which have you not?

3. How easy or difficult was it to remember where the cards were?
4. Why was it important to use good concentration skills for this game?
5. For what other activities is it important to use good concentration skills?
6. Which of the sports mentioned today would you like to learn?

**Leadership Considerations:**
1. Content of playing cards should be appropriate to group's age level.

2. The leader should make sure that everyone takes a turn at the appropriate time.

**Variations:**
1. The participants could make the playing cards.
2. The leader could alter the content of the playing cards to meet the needs of the group.

**Creator:** Kate Czerwinski, Illinois State University, Normal, Illinois.

# Sidewalk Chalk

**Space Requirements:** Classroom or activity room and outdoor area with a sidewalk

**Equipment/Resource Requirements:** Paper, markers, colored pencils, sidewalk chalk

**Group Size:** Small group

**Program Goals:**

1. To increase participants' awareness of favorable outdoor leisure activities.
2. To allow participants the opportunity to express creativity.

**Program Description:**
**Preparation:**
The leader should have supplies ready and a prepared example to share with the group.

**Introduction:**
The leader will explain to the participants that there are two steps to this activity. The first step will be done indoors and the second step outdoors. Next, the leader will discuss leisure activities, focusing on activities that are typically done outdoors.

**Activity Description:**
The leader will distribute one piece of paper to each participant. The participants will draw a picture of their favorite outdoor leisure activity. Once they complete this step, the leader will ask them to share their picture with the group and explain why they consider it to be their favorite, who taught them how to do this activity, with whom they usually do the activity, where in the outdoors they do this activity, and how often they usually do it.

Next, the group will go outside. The leader will give each person one package of sidewalk chalk and instruct the participants to replicate their drawing onto the sidewalk and then sign their name next to it. After this step is complete, the group will return to the activity room and discuss the following questions.

**Debriefing Questions/Closure:**

1. When it is warm outside, what are two other things each of you like to do?
2. What do you like to do when it is raining and you are unable to go outside?
3. Was it more difficult to draw your favorite activity on the sidewalk with the chalk or on the paper with the markers?
4. Why is this activity your favorite?
5. Do you think you'll have the same favorite activity a year from now?

**Leadership Considerations:**

1. The leader should have a discussion with the group about activities they can do outside in large groups.
2. The leader should tell the participants that what they draw on the paper will be what they draw on the sidewalk.

**Variation:**
As a group, the participants may make one large drawing of a playground or park and all of the leisure opportunities there.

**Creator:** Connie Campbell, Illinois State University, Normal, Illinois.

# Which Way Is the Wind Blowing?

**Space Requirements:** Classroom or activity room

**Equipment/Resource Requirements:** Wire coat hangers, aluminum foil, pint-size plastic tub, scissors, sand, masking tape and permanent markers

**Group Size:** Small group

**Program Goals:**
1. To increase participants' knowledge of the weather and the purpose of a weather vane.
2. To increase participants' cooperation skills by having everyone share supplies.

**Program Description:**
**Preparation:**
The leader should gather equipment and have an example completed.

**Introduction:**
This activity will allow participants to become more aware of the use of a weather vane and how the wind can predict the type of weather that may come along.

**Activity Description:**
The leader will explain what a weather vane is and how it is used. The participants then will begin constructing their own weather vane. The steps to complete this are as follows:

1. Fill the pint-size container (completely) with sand.
2. Place the lid on the container.
3. On the sides of the container, write the letters *N, S, E,* and *W* with a permanent marker.
4. Bend the wire coat hanger so that the curved top is straight.
5. Cover half of the hanger with the aluminum foil, securing the foil with tape.
6. Using the top of the hanger, make a hole in the top of the lid of the sand-filled container.
7. The hanger is now in place and the weather vane is complete.

When the wind blows, the open part of the hanger will point to the direction the wind is coming from. The foil-covered part of the hanger will point in the direction the wind is blowing toward. The leader should have the group go outside (if current weather conditions are pleasant), and place the weather vane in a safe place (where it will not blow away). As a group, the participants should determine which direction the wind is coming from and try to predict what the weather may be like in the near future.

**Debriefing Questions/Closure:**
1. In regard to your leisure lifestyle, why could it be important or necessary to know what the weather is going to be like?
2. Which of your favorite activities require a particular weather condition?
3. How else can you find out what the weather is going to be like?

**Leadership Consideration:**
The leader should have a weather vane prepared before the activity.

**Variation:**
The participants could decorate their pint-size containers.

**Creator:** Kate Czerwinski, Illinois State University, Normal, Illinois.

# Masterpiece of Imagination

**Space Requirements:** Classroom or activity room

**Equipment/Resource Requirements:** Large mixing bowl, spoon, newspaper, four small bowls, white construction paper, six tablespoons of water, one-half cup of cornstarch, and food coloring (any color)

**Group Size:** Small group

**Program Goals:**
1. To increase participants' awareness of their leisure preferences.
2. To increase participants' cooperation skills by having everyone share supplies.
3. To increase participants' ability to follow directions and remain on task.

**Program Description:**
**Preparation:**
The leader should gather supplies and set up the activity area. A completed example should be prepared to share with the group.

**Introduction:**
The main purpose of this activity is to increase participants' awareness of their leisure preferences.

**Activity Description:**
The leader will explain to the participants that they are going to express themselves through a hands-on activity. Several steps are involved in this activity. (The are described here in chronological order. The ingredient amounts are per participant.)

1. In large mixing bowl combine $1/2$ cup of cornstarch with 4 tablespoons of water. Stir until well-blended.
2. Distribute a handful of the mixed substance to each of the participants.

3. The participants will be given approximately five minutes to play with the substance. The substance should hold shape for this allotted time period. The leader should instruct the participants to create different shapes with the substance. While playing with the substance, the participants should add more water to their mixture if the substance is too crumbly. They should avoid using too much water.
4. Next, the participants will lay down newspaper at their working area.
5. The leader will gather all of the substance from the participants.
6. The leader will equally divide the substance into four small bowls.
7. The leader will add food coloring to each bowl; this creates watercolor paint. The leader may add small amounts of water as necessary.
8. The leader will distribute one piece of construction paper to each participant.
9. The leader will instruct participants to begin creating their masterpiece by using their hands and fingers to create a picture of their favorite leisure activity. The leader should encourage the use of creativity and self-expression.

**Debriefing Questions/Closure:**
1. Discuss each participant's masterpiece of imagination.
2. Have each participant explain why he or she created what he or she did.
3. How was your favorite activity the same as or different from everyone else?
4. How often do you get to participate in this activity?
5. Name two reasons why it's your favorite activity.

**Leadership Consideration:**
The leader may have some of the watercolor made ahead of time.

**Variation:**
The topic may be changed to favorite sport, typical Saturday, or dream vacation.

**Creator:** Kate Czerwinski, Illinois State University, Normal, Illinois.

# Recreation Inventory

**Space Requirements:** Classroom or activity room

**Equipment/Resource Requirements:** Blank paper, pencils

**Group Size:** Small group

**Program Goals:**
1. To increase participants' awareness of leisure resources.
2. To increase participants' awareness of leisure resources in the home.
3. To increase participants' awareness of leisure resources in the community.

**Program Description:**
**Introduction:**
The purpose of this activity is to make participants aware of the abundance of recreational resources that surround them.

**Activity Description:**
The leader will distribute two pieces of paper and a pencil to each participant. As a group, the leader and the participants will go through the following list of recreational activities:

- archery,
- baseball,
- basketball,
- biking,
- billiards/pool,
- bowling,
- canoeing,
- cards,
- cooking,
- dancing,
- drawing/art,
- fishing,
- football,
- gymnastics,
- hockey,

- miniature golf,
- Ping-Pong,
- reading,
- running,
- sewing,
- soccer,
- swimming,
- tennis, and
- volleyball.

The leader will ask each participant to write down each activity mentioned. After the entire list has been read, the leader will have each participant write down the equipment, playing area, and/or facilities needed for each activity.

Next, the leader will have each participant go back through the list of activities and write down the nearest location of each, for example:

*Swimming:*
[Equipment] Swimming Suit (drawer)
[Playing Area/Facilities] Swimming Pool (community pool)

Once this step is completed, the participants will put an *H* next to each resource that would be found in their home, and a *C* next to the resources that can be found within the community. To conclude the activity, the leader will have each participant go through his or her list and discuss the resources. The leader will focus on the fact that there are many resources located within the home and the community. The leader will encourage participants to use this list as a reference if there is ever a time that they cannot think of anything to do.

**Debriefing Questions/Closure:**
1. What kinds of resources did you need for the previous recreational activities?
2. What are two activities that you have the resources for in your home or your room?

3. What is something that you have the resources for in your town?
4. Now that you have this list completed, do you plan to participate in these activities more?

**Leadership Considerations:**
1. The leader should give a clear example to the participants, so they fully understand the activity.

2. The leader should give suggestions of where some resources of which the participants may not be aware could be found.

**Variation:**
The activity could be geared toward teamwork, and the group could work together to make a list of the resources within the agency and the community.

**Creator:** Jessica Kamm, Illinois State University, Normal, Illinois.

# Building a Park

**Space Requirements:** Classroom or activity room

**Equipment/Resource Requirements:** Play-Doh, flat working surface

**Group Size:** Small group

**Program Goals:**
1. To increase participants' awareness of facilities and resources typically found in a park.
2. To increase participants' ability to cooperate with peers in a small group situation.
3. To increase participants' ability to follow directions and remain on task.

**Program Description:**
**Introduction:**
The purpose of this activity is to increase the participants' awareness of park facilities and resources, while improving their ability to act cooperatively, follow directions and remain on task.

**Activity Description:**
The leader will give each participant a large amount of Play-Doh. The leader will explain to the participants that they will be working as a team to construct a park. The park that is to be constructed should include elements such as a lake, trees, animals, bushes, and playground equipment.

The participants will be given an appropriate time limit to complete the activity. The participants will have to decide among themselves who will take which responsibilities to construct the park. The leader should encourage the group to discuss a plan of action and to cooperate so that the park can be constructed within the time limit. When the time limit is up, the leader and the participants will discuss the activity. The discussions should include what was done well and/ or could have been done better to complete the

activity more efficiently and effectively. The leader should focus the discussion on teamwork and cooperation.

The leader should reemphasize the goals of the activity. Debriefing questions are provided below.

**Debriefing Questions/Closure:**
1. What are the most important elements of a park?
2. Why do we go to parks? What do parks offer us?
3. Describe your most positive experience at a park.
4. What was the most challenging aspect of the activity? What was the least challenging aspect?
5. How difficult was it to coordinate the entire group to complete the activity in a limited amount of time?
6. If you could do the activity again what would you suggest the group do to work in a more efficient and effective manner?

**Leadership Considerations:**
1. The leader may provide old clothes or some type of coverup shirt. This may be necessary when working with Play-Doh.
2. The leader may want to have cookie cutters or some kind of molds that the participants can use to form shapes.

**Variations:**
1. As the participants begin to work better together, the time limit could be decreased and other pieces of a park be made additional requirements in order to increase the challenge.
2. The time limit for activity completion can be increased in order to decrease the challenge if participants are lower functioning.

3. This activity could be used more than once with the same group by changing the setting that the participants are creating. Some suggested settings include a zoo, beach, or any other recreational facilities.

**Creator:** Jessica Kamm, Illinois State University, Normal, Illinois.

# What to Do on a Rainy Day

**Space Requirements:** Classroom or activity room

**Equipment/Resource Requirements:** Paper, markers, index cards, stapler

**Group Size:** Small group

**Program Goals:**
1. To increase participants' awareness of personal leisure resources.
2. To increase participants' awareness of leisure resources and activities located within the home.

**Program Description:**
**Preparation:**
A completed example should be prepared to share with the group.

**Introduction:**
This activity is designed to increase participants' awareness of resources located within the home.

**Activity Description:**
The leader will give each participant a piece of paper and instruct the participants to fold the paper in half and staple the sides. Now the paper can be used as a pouch. Next, the participants will label the pouch "My Rainy Day Activities."

The leader should initiate a discussion on leisure resources that are in the home, such as board games, arts and crafts supplies, sports equipment, and so on. Next, the participants will brainstorm leisure activities that they enjoy and can be done in the home or residence on a rainy day. These activities and resources should represent actual activities and resources that a person has or does in his or her own home.

Next, the participants will write the name of each of these leisure resources or activities on an index card. A minimum of five cards should be filled out; there is no maximum number. When each of the cards has been completed, the participant will fold it in half and put the card into the "rainy day" pouch. Now the pouch serves as a resource for a variety of activities that can be done on a rainy day. The participants can simply choose a card and have an idea ready for them.

**Debriefing Questions/Closure:**
1. What are three activities that you put on your cards?
2. What resources are needed for each?
3. Which of the activities or resources are your favorites? Why?
4. What are things you can do when you're home on a rainy day?

**Leadership Considerations:**
1. The leader should offer the participants some examples to get them brainstorming.
2. The leader should encourage the participants to make as many cards as possible in the time given in order to have more options available to them on the next rainy day.

**Variation:**
If participants are residing in a residential home, they should create a list of activities that they like to do in their free time or are available at the facility.

**Creator:** Jessica Kamm, Illinois State University, Normal, Illinois.

# Feelings Recipe Bag

**Space Requirements:** Classroom or activity room

**Equipment/Resource Requirements:** Construction paper, markers, scissors, stapler or glue, index cards, magazines (optional)

**Group Size:** Small group

**Program Goals:**
1. To increase participants' awareness of the causes of personal feelings related to leisure.
2. To increase participants' ability to explore what leisure activities elicit certain feelings for them.

**Program Description:**
**Introduction:**
This activity was designed to increase participants' awareness of their feelings toward different leisure activities.

**Activity Description:**
The leader will give each participant the needed materials and have each make a pouch out of construction paper. This is accomplished by folding the paper in half and stapling the two sides so that there is an opening at the top.

Next, the leader will explain to the participants that they are to design a picture that represents them, and put their name on the cover of the pouch. Following this, the participants will make recipe cards to go inside the pouch. On the front of each card the participants will write a feeling (one feeling per card). The following feelings are suggested: happy, excited, sad, angry, fearful, and proud.

On the other side of the index card each participant will write examples of a leisure activity or experience that caused him or her to feel this way in the past. It may be necessary to explain what leisure is. Participants can either draw the activity on the card or cut a representative picture out of a magazine. When the activity has been completed each participant can share his or her recipes with the group and discuss the reasons that these feelings may or may not have been caused.

**Debriefing Questions/Closure:**
1. In the past, have you ever considered how certain leisure activities make you feel?
2. What is your most memorable moment of the activities you were able to recall?
3. Do you associate mostly positive feelings or negative feelings with leisure? Why?
4. How can you use leisure activities to help create positive feelings?
5. What would you do if you wanted to help yourself get into a better mood?

**Leadership Considerations:**
1. The leader should have a few examples completed to share with the group.
2. The leader may have to hold a discussion on what leisure means.

**Variation:**
Focus can be placed on activities that the participants have never tried before. The participants then can describe any feelings of reluctance for the activity and/or feelings of excitement they anticipate.

**Creator:** Jessica Kamm, Illinois State University, Normal, Illinois.

# Your Magical Butterfly Can Take You There

**Space Requirements:** Classroom or activity room

**Equipment/Resource Requirements:** Paper and writing utensils

**Group Size:** Small group

**Program Goal:**
To increase participants' awareness of personal leisure preferences.

**Program Description:**
**Introduction:**
This activity was designed to increase participants' awareness of personal leisure motives and values.

**Activity Description:**
The leader will ask the participants to sit in a circle with legs crossed in a butterfly position. Once everyone is seated, the leader will distribute a packet to each individual. The packet contains five pieces of paper. Each piece of paper is labeled with a different heading. The headings should be as follows:

- The Baby Fold [name of facility],
- Normal [city in which facility is located],
- Illinois [state in which facility is located],
- USA, and
- World.

Next, the leader will explain the directions of Magical Butterfly:

Just imagine all of the neat fun and exciting things that you do or would like to do for leisure. Your Magical Butterfly can take you there. So close your eyes and get onto your own Magical Butterfly. Now fly to your most favorite place in The Baby Fold [name of facility].

At this point, the participants are to think about their favorite place in the facility. Now, the participants should draw on that piece of paper everything they are able to think of about their favorite place.

The activity continues as the group members imagine that they are on their Magical Butterfly and fly to their most ideal place in this *city, state, country,* and finally, *world.* Each person is to draw a picture of his or her most ideal or favorite place in each of the four categories.

After all five drawings have been completed, the leader will go around to each member of the group and have the participants discuss what is important about their chosen places and why they chose them over something else. When discussing places located in a distant part of the country and world, the participant and leader should focus on setting goals that could be realistically met in the future.

**Debriefing Questions/Closure:**
1. What characteristics make each of your special places special to you?
2. What characteristics differ between each of the five places?
3. What things are important to your friends in their "fun time" that are different from yours?
4. Explain why you wanted to go where you did.
5. Why did you pick those places?

**Leadership Considerations:**
1. It may be necessary for the leader to explain what leisure is.
2. When explaining the directions, the leader should give an example of a favorite place in each of the five settings.
3. The leader should encourage the participants to think about the things that are most important to them overall, not just one favorite toy or game in a room.

**Variations:**

1. The participants could ride the Magical Butterfly into the past, and discuss the times that they have been special on trips or vacations, and the things that made them special.

2. The participants could ride the Magical Butterfly into the future and create three different vacations, describing what each would include.

**Creator:** Jessica Kamm, Illinois State University, Normal, Illinois.

# Crayon Pictures of Leisure

**Space Requirements:** Classroom or activity room

**Equipment/Resource Requirements:** One piece of white drawing paper per participant, three or four boxes of crayons, one black crayon per participant, one toothpick per participant

**Group Size:** Small group

**Program Goals:**
1. To increase participants' awareness of various leisure activities.
2. To increase participants' awareness of their favorite leisure activities.

**Program Description:**
**Preparation:**
The leader should have a completed example to show to the group. The leader should take the black crayons out of the boxes of crayons.

**Introduction:**
The leader will explain to the participants that they will be doing an activity that requires some creativity.

**Activity Description:**
The participants will sit at the table. The leader will explain the directions of the activity. Using the crayons, the participants will color or scribble over the entire piece of paper so there is *no white space* showing.

After each participant has completed this step, the leader will distribute one black crayon to each person in the group. Now, using the black cray-

ons, the participants will color over the entire sheet of paper so there are *no colors* showing.

Finally, using the toothpicks, the participants will sketch (scratch) their favorite leisure or recreation activity on their sheet of paper. During the time the group is sketching, the leader should initiate a discussion on leisure activities.

**Debriefing Questions/Closure:**
1. What is your favorite leisure activity?
2. What similarities and differences were there in your favorite leisure activities and those of other group members?
3. How easy was it to select only one activity? How difficult was it?
4. What new activities did you hear about today?
5. Why are leisure activities important to us?

**Leadership Considerations:**
1. The leader may need to give examples of various leisure and recreation activities.
2. The leader should encourage the participants to exercise positive manners in sharing the crayons with each other.

**Variation:**
The content of the sketch can be changed from favorite leisure activity to positive qualities of self or picture of self.

**Creator:** Jennifer Matkowich, Illinois State University, Normal, Illinois.

# Leisure Activities on Holiday

**Space Requirements:** Classroom or activity room

**Equipment/Resource Requirements:** One piece of 4-by-10-foot white paper, crayons, markers, tape or thumb tacks, variety of decorative craft materials (i.e., cotton, construction paper, glue, and stencils)

**Group Size:** Small group

**Program Goals:**
1. To increase participants' ability to identify leisure activities appropriate to the season.
2. To increase participants' ability to express creativity.
3. To increase participants' cooperation skills through a group activity that requires sharing and equal participation.

**Program Description:**
**Preparation:**
The leader will gather the materials and place them within reach of all participants.

**Introduction:**
The leader will explain to the participants that they will be working as a team to complete a drawing together.

**Activity Description:**
The participants will sit at the table. The leader will place the large sheet of paper in front of all participants, making sure that everyone can reach it adequately. The leader will explain to the participants that they are going to work as a team to draw a holiday scene. The scene should appropriately reflect the season (summer, fall, winter, or spring) and should contain various recreational activities that are appropriate for that season.

At this point the participants should discuss and vote on a holiday scene they are all interested in drawing. If necessary, the leader can give the group different ideas. Throughout the activity the participants should effectively communicate with one another to decide who will be drawing what and try to avoid drawing duplicates.

Once the holiday scene is completed all participants should autograph the drawing. Last, the entire group should work together to hang the drawing in a location for everyone to see.

The leader should focus discussion on what participants have learned through this activity. Debriefing questions follow.

**Debriefing Questions/Closure:**
1. How did the group decide which holiday, season, and leisure activities to draw?
2. How easy was it to decide which activities to draw? How difficult was it?
3. How essential was cooperation? How essential was communication? How essential was listening? How essential was creativity?
4. What are important elements for teamwork?
5. How did you contribute to the team? What did you do to cooperate?

**Leadership Consideration:**
The leader may encourage the participants to make a list of the different things they want to include in their holiday scene and designate who will be responsible for drawing them.

**Variations:**
1. The leader can have the group pick a scene from a bag that contains a variety of different scenes.
2. The group can draw a community picture that includes the leisure and recreation resources located within that community.
2. The leader can read a poem or short story that is related to a particular holiday and have the group then draw a picture related to that.

**Creator:** Jennifer Matkowich, Illinois State University, Normal, Illinois.

# Leisure Scattergories

**Space Requirements:** Classroom or activity room

**Equipment/Resource Requirements:** Accompanying form, pens and pencils

**Group Size:** Small group

**Program Goals:**
1. To increase participants' awareness of leisure activities.
2. To encourage participants' creative thinking in a short time span.

**Program Description:**
**Preparation:**
Questions and answer sheets should be prepared ahead of time. Content of questions and answers should be appropriate to the level of group's knowledge base and understanding.

**Introduction:**
The leader will explain to the participants that they will be playing a game that involves thinking fast and being creative. The game is played by the leader asking the group a variety of questions and the group then coming up with answers to each of the questions.

**Activity Description:**
The participants will sit at the table. The leader will explain to the participants that they each will be asked a total of 15 questions. Each of the questions has a total of five answers. The first letter of the answers must begin with a set of letters that has been chosen for that particular question. For example: If asked "Name of video games," the answers must begin with the following set of letters: *A, B, C, D, E.*

The leader will distribute an answer sheet and a writing utensil to each participant. The leader should encourage the participants to be creative in their answers and to be as original as possible. Points will be distributed as follows: each time a participant comes up with an answer that no one else has, the participant will receive one point. If another person shares the same answer, both participants will cross it off their lists and neither will receive a point. The person with the most points will be declared the winner.

At this point, the leader will begin to read the questions, giving the group three to four minutes to work on each question. The answers either can be read after each question or saved until the end of the game.

**Debriefing Questions/Closure:**
1. What new leisure activities did you hear mentioned during this session?
2. How easy was it to come up with unique answers? How difficult was it?
3. Have you participated in any of the things we talked about in this activity?
4. Why was it important to use good listening skills in this activity?
5. How creative do you think you were for this activity?

**Leadership Considerations:**
1. The leader should make sure the participants are able to read and write.
2. The leader should have an example ready to share with group prior to starting.

**Variations:**
1. An alternative content can be used instead of leisure activities for questions.
2. The participants may work in small groups rather than individually.

**Creator:** Jennifer Matkowich, Illinois State University, Normal, Illinois.

# Leisure Scattergories

## Questions

Use 15 of the following questions:

1. Name an action figure.
2. Activities to do in a park.
3. Activities to do in the summer.
4. Activities to do in the fall.
5. Activities to do in the winter.
6. Activities to do in the spring.
7. Activities to do at the [name of residential facility].
8. Names of video games.
9. Activities to do outside.
10. Activities to do inside.
11. Activities to do alone.
12. Things you would see at a swimming pool.
13. Name places you could go on vacation.
14. Name things you could see at a zoo.
15. Activities to do with your family.
16. Activities that don't cost any money.
17. Sports activities to watch.
18. Activities that involve food.
19. Special events throughout the year.
20. Activities that don't require equipment.

# Leisure Scattergories

## Answer Sheet

1. A

   B

   C

   D

   E

   _____

2. F

   G

   H

   I

   J

   _____

3. K

   L

   M

   N

   O

   _____

4. P

   Q

   R

   S

   T

5. U

   V

   W

   Y

   Z

   _____

6. A

   B

   C

   D

   E

   _____

7. F

   G

   H

   I

   J

   _____

8. K

   L

   M

   N

   O

9. P

   Q

   R

   S

   T

---

10. U

    V

    W

    Y

    Z

---

11. A

    B

    C

    D

    E

---

12. F

    G

    H

    I

    J

13. K

    L

    M

    N

    O

---

14. P

    Q

    R

    S

    T

---

15. U

    V

    W

    Y

    Z

---

# Salt Art

**Space Requirements:** Classroom or activity room

**Equipment/Resource Requirements:** Paper plates, colored chalk, salt, clear containers (clear baby food jars with lids and clear McDonald's sundae cups with lids work well), Leisure Activity Awareness work sheet

**Group Size:** Small group

**Program Goals:**
1. To increase participants' knowledge of leisure activities.
2. To allow participants to design their own salt art project.
3. To increase participants' awareness of art as leisure.

**Program Description:**
**Preparation:**
The leader should make enough copies of the work sheet for each participant. The leader should make sure there are enough materials for all the participants to work with. The leader should have an example ready to share with the group.

**Introduction:**
The leader will begin the activity by having each participant individually complete the work sheet. The leader will give five to seven minutes for this. When everyone is finished, the leader will have each person discuss his or her answers. The leader will explain that all these items are things that are necessary to participate in leisure activities. One answer not listed on the work sheet is art. Art is considered a leisure activity for many people.

The leader will ask the participants to give examples of art activities that are considered leisure. Today they will do salt art. The leader will place the supplies on the table and then explain the directions.

**Activity Description:**
The leader will begin by displaying the example prepared ahead of time to the participants. The leader will explain to them that they are going to each be making their own salt art designs. The leader should remind them that if they have any questions or need help they should ask.

The leader will demonstrate to the group how to color the salt:

1. Put about $1/8$ of a cup of salt on a paper plate.
2. Take a piece of chalk and rub it back and forth (lay chalk down) on the paper plate to color the salt.
3. Pour the salt into the cup and begin again with fresh, uncolored salt.

The leader will explain that they can make the salt as light or dark as they choose. Then the leader should clarify that this process will be repeated until the container is full. At that time, a lid will be placed on the salt art design.

The leader will pass around the paper plates, salt, cups and chalk so that each participant has one to use. If there are not enough supplies, participants may share with one another. The leader should encourage the participants to begin as soon as everyone has the materials.

As the participants are finishing up, the leader should encourage them to clean up any mess that may have been made.

**Debriefing Questions/Closure:**
1. What leisure activities did you hear about today (through the work sheet)?
2. What types of art activities are considered leisure?
3. What are the benefits of art activities, such as this salt art project?
4. What other art activities would you like to learn or teach others?

**Leadership Considerations:**
1. The leader should have one box of chalk for each participant if possible.
2. The leader should encourage the participants to rub the salt slowly or it will make quite a mess.

**Variations:**
1. When using colored chalk with children, the leader may have them explain what some of the colors mean to them or how each color makes them feel (self-awareness).
2. The participants may decorate their jars to resemble people (use googly eyes, yarn for hair, pipe cleaners for body parts, and so on).
3. The leader may tie in the activity with a discussion about chores and responsibilities. The leader may have the participants be responsible for cleaning up their own mess.

**Creator:** Amanda L. McGowen, Illinois State University, Normal, Illinois.

(*Answers:* 1. football; 2. golf; 3. racquetball; 4. lacrosse; 5. tennis; 6. hockey; 7. volleyball; 8. baseball; 9. wallyball; 10. jogging; 11. badminton; 12. soccer; 13. archery; 14. swimming; 15. bowling; 16. fishing; 17. weightlifting; 18. fencing; 19. skiing; and 20. aerobics.)

# Salt Art

## Leisure Activity Awareness

*Directions:* Complete the leisure activities below by using the letter clues (which are all the vowels of the word) and the word clues to the right.

1. _ O O _ _ A _ _      Yard lines

2. _ O _ _      Clubs

3. _ A _ _ U E _ _ A _ _      Court

4. _ A _ _ O _ _ E      Long-handled stick

5. _ E _ _ I _      Racquet

6. _ O _ _ E _      Goal

7. _ O _ _ E _ _ A _ _      Net

8. _ A _ E _ A _ _      Bat

9. _ A _ _ _ _ A _ _      Walls

10. _ O _ _ I _ _      Sweats

11. _ A _ _ I _ _ O _      Birdie

12. _ O _ _ E _      Goal

13. A _ _ _ E _ _      Bow

14. _ _ I _ _ I _ _      Water

15. _ O _ _ I _ _      Lanes

16. _ I _ _ I _ _      Pole

17. _ E I _ _ _ _ I _ _ I _ _      Bench

18. _ E _ _ I _ _      Foil or saber

19. _ _ I I _ _      Snow or water

20. A E _ O _ I _ _      Leotards

Source: Stumbo, N. J. (1992). *Leisure Education II: More Activities and Resources*. State College, PA: Venture Publishing, Inc., p. 179. Reprinted with permission of Venture Publishing, Inc.

# My Day to Play

**Space Requirements:** Classroom or activity room

**Equipment/Resource Requirements:** Entertainment section of the newspaper, pieces of lined paper, writing utensils (one per each participant)

**Group Size:** Small group

**Program Goals:**
1. To increase participants' ability to make decisions related to leisure.
2. To increase participants' understanding of factors involved in making a decision.
3. To increase participants' ability to locate information about community leisure resources.

**Program Description:**
**Preparation:**
The leader should prepare a completed example to share with the group.

**Introduction:**
The leader will explain to the participants that they will be working individually to complete an activity that will increase their ability to make decisions through focusing on community resources.

**Activity Description:**
The leader will begin the activity by explaining what are the important factors involved in making decisions. The leader then will initiate a discussion related to decision making. Next, the leader will explain the directions of the activity before providing participants with an entertainment section of a newspaper.

Each individual will be responsible for preparing a schedule grid to fill in with leisure- and recreation-related activities. This grid will represent one day; the times will begin and end however the individual chooses.

Each person should locate activities occurring on the chosen date and times from the entertainment section of the newspaper (e.g., dances,

festivals, movies, and concerts). Next, he or she will write down times, location, and cost next to each activity name. Each participant will determine the total amount of money that will be needed to participate in all of the activities. He or she will determine a place to call to find out more details about a specific event and call the information center with additional questions. The participant will write down information received from the call. He or she will prioritize the activities based on cost and transportation availability.

The leader will have each participant share with the group his or her planned activities. How realistic is the plan? How likely is he or she to follow through with the plan? The leader will close with debriefing questions.

**Debriefing Questions/Closure:**
1. What did you learn from this experience?
2. Who is responsible for planning your leisure?
3. What barriers, if any, did you find kept you from participating in an activity?
4. What factors did you find to be important in making decisions?
5. How can you apply these decision-making skills to everyday life?
6. How likely are you to participate in the activities you planned?

**Leadership Considerations:**
1. The leader should consider the age of the participants.
2. The leader should consider the participants' ability to read and/or write.

**Variations:**
1. Pictures may be used for individuals who are unable to read.
2. People with learning difficulties may require pictures, a reader, and/or more direct assistance from the leader.

**Creator:** Craig W. Strohbeck, Illinois State University, Normal, Illinois.

# Leisure Jenga

**Space Requirements:** Classroom or activity room

**Equipment/Resource Requirements:** Colored Jenga game (including the die), colored game cards (see accompanying form), sturdy table

**Group Size:** Small group (four per Jenga game)

**Program Goals:**
1. To increase participants' existing self-awareness of personal goals, beliefs, values, and attitudes concerning leisure.
2. To increase participants' awareness of current leisure activities.
3. To increase participants' knowledge of how others perceive their leisure.

**Program Description:**
**Preparation:**
The leader should have the game cards prepared beforehand on the correct colored cards. Lamination will increase the durability of the cards.

**Introduction:**
The leader will explain to the participants that they are going to play Leisure Jenga. This game will help them identify their own leisure interests and those of their friends.

**Activity Description:**
The rules of the game are as follows:

1. The first person to roll a wild with the die begins the game. Play then follows to the right of that person (no more than four people per Jenga game).
2. Each person is allowed to pick any colored piece and put it on top of the pile.
3. If a player chooses to move a red Jenga piece, he or she must pick up a red Jenga card, read it and then answer it. If he or she chooses a blue Jenga piece, then he or she must answer a blue card.
4. The game continues until the Jenga pile falls or time runs out. If the pile falls and there is time for another game, the participants may start another one.

**Debriefing Questions/Closure:**
1. Name one thing that you learned about other players that you might not have known concerning their leisure interests.
2. Name one answer to a question that you liked the most and share it with the group.

**Leadership Consideration:**
If there is only one participant, a staff member could play with the participant.

**Variations:**
1. The participants could make up their own questions to add to the game.
2. The questions can relate to any content or purpose of the activity.

**Creator:** Amanda L. McGowen, Illinois State University, Normal, Illinois.

# Leisure Jenga

**Questions on Yellow Cards:**

*Goal:* To increase participants' existing self-awareness of personal goals, beliefs, values and attitudes concerning leisure.

1. Describe what you would like to do on a vacation.
2. If you had $20, what would you do with it?
3. Describe one of your favorite free-time activities.
4. What is one thing that you want to learn how to do?
5. If you could do anything for a day, what would you do?
6. What do you enjoy making in the kitchen?
7. What do you enjoy doing outside?
8. Name or describe one of your favorite parks.
9. Name one of your favorite people to spend time with.
10. What would you buy in the grocery store if you had $5?
11. Describe how you like to spend your time in the evening.
12. Name one activity that you want to try in the next year.
13. Describe what kinds of movies you enjoy watching.
14. Describe an activity that you enjoy doing alone.
15. Describe an activity that you enjoy doing in groups.

**Questions on Red Cards:**

*Goal:* To increase participants' awareness of current leisure activities.

1. Describe the types of things you like to do after school.
2. Describe what types of games you like to play with your friends.
3. Describe one of your favorite toys from when you were younger.
4. Describe your pet if you had one when you were younger.
5. Name one of your favorite songs.
6. Name one of your favorite movies.
7. Name one of your favorite TV shows.
8. Describe what you do for fun.

9. What would you like to do next Saturday?
10. Describe one of your favorite stories or books.
11. Describe what you want to be when you grow up.
12. Describe your favorite birthday present.
13. Name one of your favorite outdoor activities.
14. Name one of your favorite restaurants.
15. If you could get tickets to an event, what would it be?

**Questions on Blue Cards:**

*Goal:* To acquire knowledge of how others perceive their leisure.

1. Ask another player to describe one of his or her favorite games to play.
2. Ask another player to describe one thing that he or she could teach someone.
3. Ask another player to describe what kinds of movies he or she enjoys.
4. Ask another player to describe an activity that he or she doesn't consider leisure.
5. Ask another player to describe an activity that he or she enjoys doing alone.
6. Ask another player to describe an activity that he or she enjoys doing in groups.
7. Ask another player to describe his or her favorite restaurant.
8. Ask another player to describe his or her dream vacation.
9. Ask another player what he or she enjoys making in the kitchen.
10. Ask another player to name his or her favorite park.
11. Ask another player to name one person he or she really enjoys spending time with.
12. Ask another player to describe his or her favorite meal.
13. Ask another player to describe what he or she wants to be when he or she grows up.
14. Ask another player to describe his or her favorite birthday present.
15. Ask another player to describe what he or she would buy in the grocery store if he or she had $5.

# Leisure Draw

**Space Requirements:** Classroom or activity room

**Equipment/Resource Requirements:** Cards with examples of leisure activities, chalkboard or other material to draw on

**Group Size:** Small group

**Program Goals:**
1. To increase participants' knowledge of different leisure activities.
2. To increase participants' ability to work together as group.
3. To allow participants the opportunity to display good sportsmanship skills.

**Program Description:**
**Preparation:**
The leader should have the cards made up ahead of time with the different leisure activities on them. Examples of leisure activities to be placed on cards include:

- baseball,
- basketball,
- bowling,
- camping,
- cooking,
- dancing,
- drawing,
- exercising,
- karate,
- fishing,
- gardening,
- hiking,
- hockey,
- hunting,
- ice-skating,
- in-line skating,
- music,
- painting,
- playing tag,
- pottery or ceramics,
- reading,
- sewing,
- skiing,
- soccer,
- swimming, and
- woodworking.

**Activity Description:**
The leader will divide the participants into two groups and have them sit in two separate areas of the room, facing the drawing board. The leader will have each group decide on a number between one and one hundred to determine which team goes first (the one closest to a predetermined number chosen by the leader starts).

The leader will explain to the groups that they are going to play a leisure version of Win, Lose, or Draw. The leader will explain that one person from each group will come forward to the drawing board, pick a card, and draw the leisure activity presented on the card. The leader will explain that some may not be as easy to draw as others but each activity is something that other individuals their age enjoy as a hobby or like to do in their spare time.

Each team will get a point if the team members guess correctly and each team will have 45 seconds to guess what leisure activity the team member is drawing. If the team members are unable to correctly guess the answer, the other team will have the opportunity to guess the answer to earn the point. At the end of the game, the team that displayed the most positive sportsmanship will earn three extra points.

**Debriefing Questions/Closure:**
1. What is one leisure activity that you learned about today?
2. What is one leisure activity you would like to try in the near future?
3. Have you ever taught another individual how to do a leisure activity?

**Leadership Consideration:**

When deciding which team chooses a number for who goes first, the leader may have each participant choose a number between 1 and 10, add those numbers up, and that will be the number for the team. (If the teams are small, they may each choose between 1 and 20.)

**Variations:**

1. If there is time at the end of the game, the leader may give each person a note card to write one activity that he or she likes to do in his or her leisure. It may be one that was already named. Then, the leader will collect the cards and have the participants draw what they wrote to their own team for extra bonus points (two points for each correct answer).

2. Instead of activities, other content can be placed on the cards, e.g., leisure equipment, places to go, sports.

**Creator:** Amanda L. McGowen, Illinois State University, Normal, Illinois.

# Activity Charades

**Space Requirements:** Classroom or activity room

**Equipment/Resource Requirements:** Pen and paper to keep score, Activity Charade cards (see examples)

**Group Size:** Small group

**Program Goals:**
1. To improve participants' awareness of leisure activities.
2. To improve participants' sportsmanship skills.

**Program Description:**
**Preparation:**
The leader should have cards made up ahead of time. The content of the cards should be different leisure activities, such as:

- archery,
- basketball,
- bowling,
- cooking,
- eating ice cream,
- exercising,
- fishing,
- football,
- going to an amusement park,
- in-line skating,
- painting,
- playing catch,
- playing games,
- playing Nintendo or Sega,
- playing the piano,
- reading,
- riding a bike,
- riding a horse,
- sewing,
- shopping,
- singing,
- softball,
- swimming,
- tennis,
- volleyball, and
- watching TV.

**Introduction:**
The leader will explain to the participants that they are going to play Activity Charades. But, before playing the game, it is necessary to discuss what good sportsmanship is. The leader will go through the following discussion questions with the participants:

1. Have you ever played a game and lost by one or two points? How did that make you feel?
2. What are ways to show that you are a good sport, even if you or your team loses a game?
3. What are some ways that people show poor sportsmanship?
4. When you show good sportsmanship, how does that affect you and other people?

**Activity Description:**
The leader will divide participants into two teams. The teams will pick to see who goes first (leader can choose how this will be done).

When it is a team's turn, the team will receive a card with a leisure activity on it. One person from the team must act out the leisure activity to his or her teammates without talking. He or she will be given one minute to act out the leisure activity. During that one-minute time limit, the team members guess what their teammate is doing. If they give the correct answer, they will be given one point. If they are unable to guess the correct answer within one minute, the opposing team will be given a chance to say its guess for one point.

The leader will explain that the team that displays the most positive sportsmanship will earn an extra two points at the end. (This will be determined by the activity leader.) What the leader will be looking for is examples of sportsmanship that were discussed earlier in the activity.

**Debriefing Questions/Closure:**
1. Which activities were easiest to guess?
2. Were there any activities you hadn't heard of before?
3. How did you demonstrate good sportsmanship during this activity?
4. Discuss other situations (maybe at school) where the participants could practice good sportsmanship.

**Leadership Considerations:**
1. The leader should be sure to praise participants when they are displaying good sportsmanship.
2. The time allowed to act out the activity written on the card may be adjusted depending on the abilities of the participants.
3. The leader should remind the participants that not all of the leisure activities involve sports or playing a game. Good sportsmanship applies to all sorts of situations.

**Variation:**
The leader could have each of the participants write down an activity that he or she enjoys doing. Then the leader could have each act it out to see if his or her team can guess what it is.

**Creator:** Amanda L. McGowen, Illinois State University, Normal, Illinois.

# Leisure Jeopardy

**Space Requirements:** Classroom or activity room

**Equipment/Resource Requirements:** Twenty-five note cards, five pieces of blank paper, one score sheet, one writing utensil, tape, a large surface (such as a wall) to hang note cards on, two or three different materials that make noise (i.e., bell, whistle, buzzer), time keeping device

**Group Size:** Small group

**Program Goal:**
To increase participants' ability to recognize leisure resources at home, at school, and in the community.

**Program Description:**
**Preparation:**
Prior to the activity, the leader will do the following:

- Determine five categories of leisure resources on which to focus questions, i.e., community, state, city, school, and home.
- Create one "Final Jeopardy" answer.
- Create five "answers" for each leisure resource category.
- Write one "answer" on each note card.
- Divide the cards according to category.
- Progressively value the five cards in each category as $100, $200, $300, $400, and $500 and label the monetary value on the side of the card opposite the "answer."
- Hang the note cards (on the wall) by category in descending dollar value with $100 at the top and $500 on the bottom.
- Label the five blank pieces of paper, each with a different category name. Place these labels above their corresponding row of "answers."

**Introduction:**
The purpose of this activity is to expose participants to a variety of leisure resources and increase their ability to recognize leisure resources. Good listening skills will be necessary in order to create questions about leisure resources related to the answers.

**Activity Description:**
The leader will begin by dividing the group into teams. Each team should have no more than five participants. Next, the leader will initiate a discussion on leisure resources and provide several examples of various leisure resources. Then the leader will begin the game by determining which team will go first. This can be accomplished by picking numbers or another method. Each team will be given a noisemaker.

The team that won the opportunity to go first will chose a category and dollar value. The leader then gives the answer. At this point, the question is open to whichever team rings in first. The team responding first is allowed 20 seconds to provide a question. For example, if the answer is, "Books & Magazines," the team might reply by asking, "What leisure resources are available at the library?"

If the question is incorrect, the turn goes to the second team that rang in. This team is given the same conditions to respond. Once the correct question is given, the leader gives control of the next turn to the team that answered correctly, or in the case of no correct question, to the last team to have control. The team giving the correct question receives the dollar value indicated on the card.

Once all the "answers" have been given, the leader totals the points for each team and tells them their scores. To end the game, the leader gives a "Final Jeopardy" answer in which all teams have one minute to respond. Prior to being given the answer, they must place a wager on their response. Last, the leader declares the team with the highest dollar value at the end as the winner.

*Note:* Discussion may occur following each round to clarify information or for questions which would help the participants to better understand the topic.

**Debriefing Questions/Closure:**

1. What resources were easiest to come up with a question? What resources were most difficult?
2. What resources had you never heard of prior to this activity?
3. What are some other resources you can think of which you would include in this game?
4. What did you learn from this activity?
5. How did you need to change your listening skills in order to answer the questions correctly?

**Leadership Considerations:**

1. The leader should limit team size to five players to maintain control of each group.
2. The leader should use age-appropriate questions and resources.
3. The leader should use local or community leisure resources (i.e., Children: This park in Bloomington has a zoo. Answer: What is Miller Park?).
4. The leader should consider the mental aptitude of the participants.
5. The leader should provide answers with only one possible question.
6. The leader should have each person in the group take turns providing the questions.

**Variation:**

The content may be altered by using other categories; i.e., social skills or team-building skills or a combination of many.

**Creator:** Craig W. Strohbeck, Illinois State University, Normal, Illinois.

# Star Light, Star Bright, What Kind of Activities Do I Like?

**Space Requirements:** Classroom or activity room

**Equipment/Resource Requirements:** Various sizes of star stencils to be used for tracing (four or five different sizes), white poster board (one per participant), scissors, pencils, markers, crayons, paints, glitter

**Group Size:** Small group

**Program Goals:**
1. To increase participants' awareness of their current leisure activities.
2. To increase participants' awareness of their desired leisure activities.

**Program Description:**
**Preparation:**
Star stencils should be made ahead of time.

**Introduction:**
The leader will explain to the participants that they will be doing an activity that will allow them the opportunity to be creative. The activity will focus on describing their current leisure lifestyle. At this time, it may be necessary for the leader to explain what leisure is and what a leisure lifestyle is. It may also be helpful to give examples of various leisure activities, both traditional and nontraditional.

**Activity Description:**
The leader will place the supplies on the table, within reach of all participants. The participants will trace several stars onto their poster board. After they have traced as many stars as possible, they should then cut out the star shapes. *Note:* The number of stars should be an even number (i.e., six, eight, ten).

Next, the leader will have the participants divide their stars into two even piles. The leader will explain to the participants that they will now decorate the stars. One set of stars should represent current leisure activities they like to do and participate in frequently. The other set of stars should represent leisure activities that they would like to do, but do not currently participate in. The leader should encourage the participants to be creative in decorating their stars. They can draw pictures to represent the leisure activities, write the activity name out, or a combination of both.

The participants should be given 30–45 minutes to complete the activity. The leader will conclude the activity by having each participant share his or her set of stars with the group and explain what he or she chose to write on his or her stars and the reasons why.

The leader will refocus on the activity goals. The following debriefing questions are provided for closure.

**Debriefing Questions/Closure:**
1. How did you feel about the results of your stars?
2. What new leisure activities did you learn about as a result of participating in this activity?
3. What barriers do you have that prevent you from participating in the activities that you would like to?
4. What can you do to overcome these barriers?

**Leadership Considerations:**
1. It may not be necessary to use an even number of stars for each of the piles. The leader should give the participants the freedom to choose how many stars they want to use for each of the two categories.
2. The leader should encourage the participants to use positive, healthy leisure activities.

**Variations:**

1. The leader may tie this in with leisure resources. The participants may include on their stars the equipment or supplies needed to participate in the leisure activity or where they can engage in this activity in the community.
2. The participants may include the person or people with whom they usually participate in this activity.
3. The participants may hang their stars from a coat hanger, with fishing line or colorful yarn, to create a mobile.
4. The participants may trace the outer edges of the stars with two different colors (silver and gold) so that they are able to differentiate between current leisure activities and desired future leisure activities.

**Creator:** Lazheta Thomas, Illinois State University, Normal, Illinois.

# Leisure Olympics

**Space Requirements:** Gymnasium or large playing area

**Equipment/Resource Requirements:** Basketball, tennis ball and racquet, football helmet, football, baseball bat and ball, Hula-Hoop, tumbling mat, jump rope, stopwatch or clock, stickers and certificates to be given as awards, marker

**Group Size:** Small group

**Program Goals:**
1. To increase participants' knowledge of various types of recreational activities.
2. To increase participants' exposure to skills required in various recreational activities.

**Program Description:**
**Preparation:**
Prior to the start of the activity, the leader should set up the large playing area. Each piece of equipment should be placed around the gym or play area as an individual station. Depending on the amount of equipment available, the number of stations will vary. For example, the leader may have a tumbling station, tennis station, baseball station, football station, and a basketball station. The leader may construct stations however he or she wishes. The leader should be sure to leave a good amount of space between each station so that participants do not interfere with one another and it is a safe environment.

**Introduction:**
The purpose of this activity is to introduce the participants to a variety of recreational alternatives and experience various types of recreational opportunities. The leader will explain the purpose and procedures to the group before starting the activity. A suggestion for an introduction is as follows:

Welcome to the Leisure Olympics! Today you will prove how well each of you can utilize the equipment placed around the room, and you will be timed for your performance. You do not want to rush, but try to get through the course as quickly as possible. Each participant will get two turns and the fastest time will be the one that is recorded. At the end of the activity each person will receive a certificate of participation and a sticker. Good Luck!

**Activity Description:**
The leader will ask the participants to sit in a single file line at the beginning of the course. The leader may want to use some type of a system for arranging the participants in line.

The first participant then will be asked to stand up and on the signal to start will begin with the first station. The leader will be timing the participant's actions and record his or her time at the end of the course. The person then will go to the end of the single file line and sit down until all participants have completed the course. Some examples of station ideas are as follows:

- basketball—have the participant shoot three baskets;
- baseball—have the participant hit a baseball across the gym; and
- jump rope—have the participant jump 10–15 times.

Once each player has had one turn, the leader will read his or her time and have the participants go through the course one more time. At the end, the leader will have an awards ceremony and have each participant receive a certificate with his or her time listed on it and a sticker.

**Debriefing Questions/Closure:**
1. Did anyone's time increase during the second try?
2. How did having a time limit make you feel about your performance?
3. If you would not have been timed, do you think you would get through the course better or worse?
4. How did it feel to receive an award for your efforts?
5. How many of these activities have you tried before?
6. Which recreation skills did you already have?
7. In which of these activities would you like to continue to participate?

**Leadership Considerations:**
1. The leader should know the physical abilities of the participants, some may be slower than others. Activities should be selected in which all participants may be successful.
2. The leader should make sure to encourage the participants while they are completing the course.
3. The leader should use other staff to help with the stations.
4. The leader may want to have the group do some warmup exercise beforehand.

**Variations:**
1. The participants may go through the course once not timed and then timed the second time around.
2. The participants may be actively involved in another activity while waiting.

**Creator:** Amy Conron, Illinois State University, Normal, Illinois.

# Who Are You?

**Space Requirements:** Classroom or activity room

**Equipment/Resource Requirements:** Accompanying form, pens and pencils

**Group Size:** Small group

**Program Goals:**
1. To increase participants' awareness of self in relation to leisure.
2. To increase participants' ability to follow directions and remain on task.

**Program Description:**
**Preparation:**
Copies should be made of the Who Are You? work sheet, one per participant.

**Introduction:**
The leader will explain to the participants that they will be participating in an activity that will allow them to explore themselves and look closely at favorable leisure activities. At this time it may be necessary to discuss what leisure is and give various examples of leisure activities.

**Activity Description:**
The leader will distribute one work sheet and writing utensil to each participant. The participants and the leader, as a group, will read through the work sheets to make sure that each person understands each question. Next, the participants will answer each question by writing either *Y* for yes, *N* for no, or *M* for maybe next to each question. The leader should encourage the participants to be honest in their answers.

After the participants answer each question, they will write a paragraph or draw pictures of how they see themselves in other leisure pursuits,

examples that were not included on the work sheet. The leader will conclude the activity by having each person share his or her answers with the group, then discuss the following questions.

**Debriefing Questions/Closure:**
1. What, if anything, did you learn about yourselves from this activity?
2. How satisfied are you with your current leisure activities? What is one thing you would like to change?
3. What is one leisure activity that you will make an effort to try out in the next six months?
4. What was the most fascinating thing you learned about another individual today?

**Leadership Considerations:**
1. The leader should make sure all participants know and understand that everyone's answers may not be the same because everyone is unique in his or her own ways.
2. The questions should be made appropriate to participants' age level.
3. The leader should encourage the participants to support and accept each other's answers.

**Variations:**
1. The content of the questions may be altered.
2. The leader may choose to leave blank spaces for participants to write in their own statements about themselves.
3. The participants may act as reporters and interview another individual in the group.

**Creator:** Kate Czerwinski, Illinois State University, Normal, Illinois.

# Who Are You?

1.  Someone who likes sports?

2.  Someone who likes to sing in the shower?

3.  Someone who likes scary movies?

4.  Someone who likes hugs?

5.  Someone who gets bored easily?

6.  Someone who will watch a lot of television when you're older?

7.  Someone who likes to bike ride?

8.  Someone who likes to be alone?

9.  Someone who likes to help others when they need help?

10. Someone who likes to camp?

11. Someone who likes to take walks?

12. Someone who enjoys going to school?

13. Someone who would like to fly an airplane?

14. Someone who would like to jump out of an airplane?

15. Someone who would like to ride a horse?

16. Someone who likes to be with friends?

17. Someone who is good at art?

18. Someone who has musical talent?

19. Someone willing to learn new things?

20. Someone who will travel the world?

21. Someone who will drive a sports car?

22. Someone who likes computer games?

23. Someone who can always be counted on by his or her friends?

24. Someone who is fun to be with?

25. Someone who enjoys the outdoors?

# Leisure Pictionary

**Space Requirements:** Classroom or activity room

**Equipment/Resource Requirements:** Chalkboard or dry erase board or large pad of paper on the wall; chalk or markers; index cards with activities written on them; stopwatch

**Group Size:** Small group

**Program Goals:**
1. To increase participants' ability to identify leisure opportunities.
2. To increase participants' ability to problem solve.
3. To increase participants' ability to cooperate on a team while competing with another team.

**Program Description:**
**Preparation:**
The leader should create all of the index cards with the objects the participants will be drawing ahead of time.

**Introduction:**
The purpose of this activity is to allow each participant the opportunity to practice communication skills, to problem solve, and to increase his or her ability to identify leisure opportunities. The leader can begin the activity by asking the group if anyone has ever played Win, Lose or Draw or Pictionary. The leader then will describe the activity, making sure that everyone has a complete understanding.

**Activity Description:**
The leader will divide the participants into two teams. A player from the first team will stand in front of both teams, next to the drawing board and read silently what is written on his or her index card. On the signal to start, the player will have 90 seconds to draw what he or she read on the card. The leader will be responsible for keeping track of time.

Only the current player's team members are allowed to guess what their teammate is drawing. If the team correctly guesses what the player is drawing, the team receives a point. If the team does not guess correctly, the turn is handed over to the other team and the other team has a chance to guess what the drawing is. If the other team guesses correctly, the other team receives a point.

Once the first team has taken its turn, a player from the second team comes to the front and the process is repeated. The game is played until all players have had a turn to draw, or until time runs out.

The leader will end this activity with a review of the purpose and goals. The following are several debriefing questions.

**Debriefing Questions/Closure:**
1. With which of the activities were you familiar? With which were you not familiar?
2. Which of these activities can you do well?
3. Which do you want to learn?
4. What was the easiest part of this activity? What was the most difficult?
5. Name one of the activities in which you will participate this week.

**Leadership Considerations:**
1. The leader should be aware of how well the participants work in group activities.
2. The leader should have a variety of activities for participants to draw.
3. The leader should make sure all the players get a chance to draw.

4. The leader should use content that the participants are familiar with and is at their ability level.

**Variations:**
1. This game may be turned into a charades (acting out) game.

2. The leader may choose to use additional types of categories, other than leisure and recreation.

**Creator:** Amy Conron, Illinois State University, Normal, Illinois.

# Leisure Charades

**Space Requirements:** Classroom or activity room

**Equipment/Resource Requirements:** Index cards with different words or phrases the participants will act out

**Group Size:** Small group

**Program Goals:**
1. To increase participants' awareness of a variety of traditional and nontraditional leisure activities.
2. To increase participants' cooperation skills.
3. To allow participants the opportunity to act out activities creatively.

**Program Description:**
**Preparation:**
The leader should determine ahead of time what cards the participants will use for the game. Some suggested scenarios are as follows:

- canoeing down a river,
- doll collecting,
- eating at a restaurant,
- fishing,
- gardening with a rake,
- going down a slide,
- going on a picnic,
- going on vacation,
- going to the circus,
- kicking a soccer ball,
- making cookies,
- playing a piano,
- playing baseball,
- playing computer games,
- playing miniature golf,
- playing volleyball,
- reading a book,
- riding a bike,
- shopping,
- skateboarding,
- surfing the Internet,
- talking on the telephone,
- watching television, and
- watching a movie.

**Introduction:**
The purpose of this activity is to allow each participant to act out creatively, demonstrate cooperation skills, and become acquainted with a variety of traditional and nontraditional leisure activities.

It is suggested to begin the activity with an introduction similar to the following:

Today we are going to act out a variety of leisure-related scenarios without using any verbal communication. It will be your job to guess what your teammates are trying to tell you. Pay close attention and say whatever activity comes to your mind.

**Activity Description:**
The leader will begin the activity by dividing the players into two teams. To start, the leader will ask one player from the first team to come up and read silently what is on the card. That person then will act out the scenario on the card. Players from his or her team will guess what he or she is acting out. Each person will be given one minute to act out. After the one-minute time limit, if the correct answer has not been reached, the participants on the opposing team may take a guess. When a team guesses the correct answer, it receives one point.

The conclusion of the game will come when all the cards have been acted out or time runs out. The winning team will be the one with the most points.

The leader should close the activity by refocusing on the goals. The following debriefing questions can facilitate discussion.

**Debriefing Questions/Closure:**

1. What new activities did you hear about today?
2. In which of these activities have you participated? In which of these activities have you not participated?
3. What new leisure activities would you like to learn?
4. How difficult was it to guess what the person was acting out?
5. What did you learn from this activity?
6. How can you use this information in the future?

**Leadership Considerations:**

1. The leader should know how well his or her participants work in a team situation.

2. The leader should know if his or her participants can handle competition.
3. The leader should assist the participants in reading the cards if necessary.

**Variations:**

1. Instead of having two teams, the leader may choose to have each person compete on his or her own. Each person can act out his or her scenario in front of the entire group and if someone from the group guesses correctly, the individual then gets a point.
2. This may be played as a Win, Lose or Draw game.
3. The content of the game may be altered to something other than leisure activities.

**Creator:** Amy Conron, Illinois State University, Normal, Illinois.

# Sports Collage

**Space Requirements:** Classroom or activity room

**Equipment/Resource Requirements:** Several sport magazines, glue or glue sticks, small poster board or construction paper, scissors

**Group Size:** Small group

**Program Goal:**
To increase participants' knowledge of sports.

**Program Description:**
**Preparation:**
The leader will randomly lay out all of the supplies on a table. The leader may choose to create a personal collage to show as a completed example to the group.

**Introduction:**
The purpose of this activity is to increase participants' knowledge of sports. The leader begins by explaining the purpose of the activity and initiating a discussion on sports.

A suggestion for beginning the activity is as follows:

How many people like sports? What kinds of sports do you enjoy playing or watching, and who are some of your favorite sports figures? Today we are going to make a collage of sports; it can include your favorite sports and sports heroes. After you have completed the collage we are going to discuss our pictures.

**Activity Description:**
The leader should explain to the participants what a collage is and perhaps show the completed example. The participants will choose and cut out different pictures from the magazines that they want to include in their collage and then glue the pictures onto the piece of paper they have been given.

Once all the group members have completed their collage, the leader will have them describe what types of pictures they have on their paper and why they put them there.

**Debriefing Questions/Closure:**
1. Why did you choose the pictures you pasted on your collage?
2. What is your favorite sport to play?
3. Where do you play the sport?
4. Who is your favorite sports hero?
5. Tell us all about your picture and why it is important to you.

**Leadership Considerations:**
1. The leader should find out ahead of time whether his or her group has an interest in sports.
2. The leader should not force anyone to participate in the activity.

**Variations:**
1. The group, as a whole, can create one large collage of sports on a large piece of poster board.
2. The leader may choose a completely different collage theme with the participants, i.e., gardening, famous people, vacation spots, or a collage "all about me."
3. The leader may encourage participants to draw pictures on their collage.

**Creator:** Amy Conron, Illinois State University, Normal, Illinois.

# My Leisure Ad

**Space Requirements:** Activity room

**Equipment/Resource Requirements:** Glue, scissors, magazines, markers, white poster board

**Group Size:** Small group

**Program Goals:**
1. To increase participants' understanding of past, present, and future nonusing leisure activities.
2. To increase participants' awareness of leisure activities that are nonusing.
3. To enable participants to increase self-disclosure in a large group setting.

**Program Description:**
**Preparation:**
The leader should gather and set out materials. The leader should prepare an example for demonstration.

**Introduction:**
The leader will explain the purpose of the activity. The major goal of this activity is to explore constructive, nonusing activities available in leisure. Before starting the activity, the leader will discuss the importance of leisure in life, now and in the future.

**Activity Description:**
The leader will have participants sit anywhere they are comfortable. All participants will have one piece of poster board to work with. The ad can be designed any way they wish as long as it represents past, present, and future nonusing leisure activities. Participants can cut items or words from magazines or draw leisure activities that are nonusing.

The leader should give the participants 20 to 30 minutes for completion. The leader will assist and answer any questions.

When the ads are completed, individuals should share their ads with the group. Discussion should focus on why leisure has changed or stayed the same throughout life and how it will change or stay the same in the future. The following discussion and debriefing questions can help refocus on the goals of the activity.

Once the activity is complete the leader will thank the group members for participating and ask them to help clean up.

**Debriefing Questions/Closure:**
1. Name three nonusing leisure activities that you would like to do this week.
2. How did using affect your leisure? How did using affect your friends?
3. What are the benefits to sober leisure?
4. What are three activities you'd like to learn about in the next year?
5. How will you go about learning these activities?
6. What does your ad say about your leisure or your attitude toward leisure?

**Leadership Considerations:**
1. The leader should be sure participants are choosing future leisure activities that are nonusing.
2. The leader should provide an example of an ad and how to present it to the group.
3. If some participants finish before others, the leader will discuss their ad with them ahead of time.

**Variations:**
1. The leader could have participants focus only on future leisure and why it is important.
2. Participants could work in groups of two or three and create a future leisure mural.

**Creator:** Lisa Koerner, Illinois State University, Normal, Illinois.

# Draw That Resource

**Space Requirements:** Activity room

**Equipment/Resource Requirements:** List of leisure activities, dry erase board and markers, timer

**Group Size:** Small group

**Program Goals:**
1. To increase participant's ability to identify a variety of activity opportunities available to them in the community.
2. To increase participants' ability to identify leisure resources within the facility, home and community.

**Program Description:**
**Preparation:**
The leader will gather supplies and prepare a list of leisure activities.

**Introduction:**
The leader will state the goals and the purpose of the activity and discuss available leisure resources in the home, agency, and/or community. The leader will divide the group into groups of three. The game used is Pictionary or drawing charades.

**Activity Description:**
This activity utilizes three categories of leisure resources: home resources, facility resources, and community resources. Groups will choose a piece of paper from a hat. Whichever resource is picked is the one the group must draw. The leader will have a list of resources for each category (see examples) and will choose which one the participant will draw. Possible resources include:

*Home leisure resources:*
- basement,
- board games,
- books,
- computer,
- kitchen,
- pets,
- plants,
- stereo or CD player,
- television, and
- yard;

*Facility leisure resources:*
- activity area,
- art supplies,
- games closet,
- garden,
- gym area,
- library,
- play area,
- puzzles,
- radio,
- sports equipment,
- television, and
- toy chest;

*Community leisure resources:*
- baseball diamond,
- climbing wall,
- lake,
- library,
- museum,
- park,
- playing fields,
- shopping mall,
- soccer field,
- swimming pool,
- trail or hiking path, and
- zoo.

Each person may pass one time and be given another resource to draw. Five points for each picture guessed within one minute will be given to the team with the correct guess. The winning team is the group with the most points.

The leader will conclude with a discussion of importance of knowing the different types of leisure resources.

**Debriefing Questions/Closure:**

1. Name three leisure resources you have in your home that you can use for leisure.
2. Name three leisure resources that are here in this facility that you can use for leisure.
3. Name three leisure resources that are in the community that you can use for leisure.
4. Why is it important to be aware of the leisure resources around you?

**Leadership Considerations:**

1. The leader will provide an example of what is meant by leisure resources before the activity begins (see examples).
2. The leader will create a list of as many community, facility, and home resources and activity opportunities available before implementing activity (see examples).

**Variation:**

The leader may want to provide more cards and have each player draw from one category; the number of points depends on how many pictures are completed in one minute.

**Creator:** Lisa Koerner, Illinois State University, Normal, Illinois.

# Leisure Benefits

**Space Requirements:** Activity room

**Equipment/Resource Requirements:** Paper, pencils, dry erase marker, dry erase board, dice

**Group Size:** Small group

**Program Goals:**
1. To increase participants' awareness of potential benefits of leisure.
2. To increase participants' cooperation in a small group setting.

**Program Description:**
**Preparation:**
The leader should gather materials and prepare an example.

**Introduction:**
The leader will explain the purpose of the activity. The major goal is to improve participants' awareness of the benefits of leisure participation. The leader will divide the participants into groups of three.

**Activity Description:**
The leader will explain to the participants that they will be brainstorming possible benefits of different leisure activities. To begin the activity the leader will ask the participants to brainstorm a list of leisure activities they enjoy, which will be written and numbered on the board. The numbers represent the number rolled using the dice so the list can only be as long as the number of dice; for example, one die equals up to six activities, two dice can accommodate 12 activities, and so on.

Group 1 will begin by rolling the dice. Whatever number Group 1 receives will be the leisure activity the group members will be working with. Each group is given one minute to list as many benefits of that activity as possible.

Each group then will name the benefits the group members listed. If any other group has the same benefit everyone must cross it off his or her list. The group with the most benefits that were not crossed off wins. Game continues until time is up (no longer than 45 minutes).

After each turn the leader will discuss the benefits listed and add more to those listed by the participants. Debriefing questions follow.

**Debriefing Questions/Closure:**
1. For which activities were benefits the easiest to identify?
2. What are some physical benefits of activities? What are some social benefits?
3. In what activities do you participate for physical benefits? In what activities do you participate for social benefits? In what activities do you participate for intellectual benefits? In what activities do you participate for emotional benefits?
4. What would happen if you never took time for leisure?
5. How can leisure help you in your daily life?

**Leadership Considerations:**
1. The leader should be prepared with some examples of leisure benefits.
2. The leader should make sure participants understand that benefits are individual to the person.

**Variations:**
1. The leader may provide a list of leisure activities at the start of the activity.
2. Each individual may list benefits rather than working in a group.

**Creator:** Lisa Koerner, Illinois State University, Normal, Illinois.

# My Piece of the Leisure Puzzle

**Space Requirements:** Activity room

**Equipment/Resource Requirements:** Large paper cut into puzzle-like pieces, scissors, tape, stencils, variety of colored markers

**Group Size:** Small group

**Program Goals:**
1. To increase participants' awareness of personal leisure preferences.
2. To increase participants' awareness of others' leisure preferences.

**Program Description:**
**Preparation:**
The leader will gather supplies and cut puzzle pieces from large sheet of paper, one piece per person.

**Introduction:**
The purpose of this activity is to increase participants' awareness of their own and others' leisure preferences. They will discuss why each person has individual preferences.

**Activity Description:**
The leader will begin by stating the purpose of the activity. Each participant will have his or her own piece of the puzzle in which he or she can draw his or her leisure preferences. Each individual should identify one or two favorite leisure activities. Participants will be given about 30 minutes to complete, if needed. Upon completion the group will use the tape to put the puzzle together on the wall.

Discussion then should focus on the variations between the pieces. Also participants can try and guess if they know what all the pieces represent.

The leader should allow the participants to discover differences as the pieces are discussed. The leader should use the debriefing questions for closure.

**Debriefing Questions/Closure:**
1. What are your favorite leisure activities?
2. How are your preferences similar to others?
3. How are your preferences different from others?
4. Why are we each unique in our preferences?
5. Why is it important to know your preferences?
6. How do you think your leisure will change over the next year? How do you think your leisure will change over the next two years?

**Leadership Considerations:**
1. The leader will precut pieces to make the puzzle mural.
2. The leader may want to make his or her own piece of the puzzle to provide an example, and also to make himself or herself more a part of the group.

**Variations:**
1. The leader could have group members create a collage of personal leisure instead.
2. The leader may want to use magazine cutouts or other art materials besides markers.

**Creator:** Lisa Koerner, Illinois State University, Normal, Illinois.

# Leisure Hangman

**Space Requirements:** Activity room

**Equipment/Resource Requirements:** List of community resources (see examples), dry erase marker and board

**Group Size:** Small group

**Program Goals:**
1. To increase participants' awareness of different community resources available for leisure participation.
2. To increase participants' competitive skills in small group setting.

**Program Description:**

**Preparation:**
The leader will prepare lists of words with a specified number of characters (see sample suggestions).

**Introduction:**
The leader will begin by stating the purpose of the activity and demonstrating an example for participants to view.

**Activity Description:**
The leader will divide the group into groups of three or four people.

There will be two categories of words from which to choose. There will be 5- and 10-point categories. The participants will be able to choose which point category from which they want a word. The different points represent the length of words. Words with 10 characters or less equal 5 points and words with 11–15 characters equal 10 points. Words with 10 or less characters include:

- aquarium,
- arcade,
- art gallery,
- camp,
- library,
- museum,
- park,
- petting zoo,
- playground,
- race track,
- restaurant,
- trail, and
- zoo.

Words with 11–15 characters include:

- amusement park,
- baseball diamond,
- community center,
- fitness center,
- movie theatre,
- nature trail,
- shopping mall,
- swimming pool, and
- tennis court.

The game will begin by having Group 1 pick the point category. The participants then begin by choosing letters. For each wrong letter the leader will begin drawing the "Hangman." If Group 1 picks a wrong letter, Group 2 will select a letter and so on. The team that guesses the word receives the point total chosen by the starting group. If Hangman is drawn, no point is given to either group.

The team with the most points is the winner. The leader will end the activity by discussing the community resources listed during the activity. The leader should use the following debriefing questions.

**Debriefing Questions/Closure:**
1. What are three community resources that you are familiar with?
2. What are three community resources that you had never heard of?

3. Name one community resource not on the list.
4. What is your favorite community resource?

**Leadership Consideration:**
If a longer word is chosen, the leader may allow more wrong answers by adding details to the Hangman such as a hat, shoes, and eyes.

**Variations:**
1. The leader could use the Wheel of Fortune rules instead of Hangman.
2. If all participants are from the same community, the leader should use actual resource names instead of general ones.

**Creator:** Lisa Koerner, Illinois State University, Normal, Illinois.

# Why Can't I Have Leisure?

**Space Requirements:** Classroom or activity room

**Equipment/Resource Requirements:** Bulletin board, paper, crayons, pens, markers, tape or stapler

**Group Size:** Small group

**Program Goals:**
1. To increase participants' awareness of leisure barriers.
2. To increase participants' awareness of removing or reducing leisure barriers.

**Program Description:**
**Preparation:**
The leader will gather supplies. Depending on level of the participants, the leader may need to prepare an initial list of leisure barriers (see examples).

**Introduction:**
The purpose of this activity is to help participants identify barriers to their independent leisure as well as ways to reduce or remove these barriers. The leader will begin the discussion by defining a leisure barrier. Typical leisure barriers include:

- attitude that leisure is not important;
- inability to get along with others;
- inability to make leisure a priority;
- lack of equipment;
- lack of money;
- lack of someone to do the activity with;
- lack of time;
- not knowing activity options;
- not knowing where to go to learn the skill;
- not knowing where to go to participate; and
- unskilled at the activity.

**Activity Description:**
The leader will give each participant a piece of paper and have available the markers, crayons and pens on a table. The leader then will tell the participants to think of what stops them from pursuing their leisure interests or activities. The participants will then create a picture of leisure barriers on the paper given. After 25 minutes, or as time allows, the leader will have the participants sit in a circle. The participants will discuss what they have created and what they could do to get around the barrier. After the discussion is completed, the leader will help the participants to place their drawings on the bulletin board with the tape or stapler provided.

Discussion should focus on what prevents them from participating in the leisure activities of their choice, and ways to remove or reduce those barriers. Closure can be aided with the following debriefing questions.

**Debriefing Questions/Closure:**
1. What is a leisure barrier?
2. What were some leisure barriers common to the group?
3. What were some unique leisure barriers identified by only one or two group members?
4. What are some ways to reduce or remove barriers to your leisure?
5. How important is attitude in removing these barriers?

**Leadership Consideration:**
Participants who have tendencies to do bodily harm should be supervised with the staples.

**Variations:**
1. The activity could use favorite leisure activities instead of leisure barriers.

2. This activity can be modified to a discussion and the leader can place the ideas in handwriting after the group meeting.
3. The activity can also use magazine cutouts to place on the paper, if desired.

**Creator:** Julie Harvey, Illinois State University, Normal, Illinois.

# Recreational Grab Bag

**Space Requirements:** Classroom or activity room

**Equipment/Resource Requirements:** Large bag, recreational equipment (any will work such as tennis balls, basketball, bat, or Ping-Pong paddle)

**Group Size:** Small group

**Program Goals:**
1. To increase participants' awareness of recreational equipment.
2. To increase participants' understanding of the uses of recreational equipment.

**Program Description:**
**Preparation:**
The leader will gather a variety of recreation equipment and place the equipment in a large bag.

**Introduction:**
The purpose of Recreational Grab Bag is to develop awareness of recreational equipment. Each object also will be demonstrated to clarify the purpose of the object.

**Activity Description:**
Each participant will sit on the floor in a circle. The leader will be in the middle with the bag filled with recreational equipment. The leader will call on a participant to come and pull out one object. The participant will then get the opportunity to name the game the object belongs to. If the participant cannot name the activity, the leader will then ask if anyone else can. The leader then will ask for a volunteer to demonstrate how the ob-

ject works. If no one can answer or act out how the object is used the leader then will do so.

After each of the participants' turn they will return the object to the leader. At the end of the activity the leader then will review each object and function with both question and answer or allowing the participants to point to the object called.

The leader should focus on the purpose of the activity and conclude with the following debriefing questions.

**Debriefing Questions/Closure:**
1. Which of the pieces of equipment do you own?
2. Which pieces were familiar to you?
3. Which pieces were new to you?
4. What leisure activity do you participate in that requires equipment?
5. What leisure activity do you participate in that does not require equipment?

**Leadership Consideration:**
Leaders should always watch demonstrations in case the participants are likely to injure themselves.

**Variations:**
1. The activity can be modified to just showing and naming the recreational equipment.
2. The activity also can be advanced and the leader can ask the participants where they can participate in the activity.

**Creator:** Julie Harvey, Illinois State University, Normal, Illinois.

# The Magic of Free Time, Me Time

**Space Requirements:** Classroom or activity room

**Equipment/Resource Requirements:** A decorated box, pictures of many different leisure activities, paper for all participants, glue or tape, scissors

**Group Size:** Small group

**Program Goals:**
1. To improve participants' awareness of their personal leisure interests.
2. To improve participants' ability to respect others' choices and use appropriate social interaction.

**Program Description:**
**Preparation:**
The leader should cut pictures of leisure activities out of magazines. The leader should have five to six pictures per participant.

**Introduction:**
The purpose of this activity is to provide participants with the opportunity to express personal leisure activity preferences and improve understanding of other group members and their unique interests.

**Activity Description:**
The leader begins by stating the goals and the purpose of the activity. The leader will instruct participants of the directions and explain that each group member must wait patiently while the other group members are taking their turns. Each participant will reach into the magic box and remove one picture. He or she has the option to keep the picture for his or her own or to pass, depending on whether he or she has ever participated in the activity or wants to someday. The participants will then be instructed to glue or tape the picture on their collage.

After all the pictures are distributed the participants will take turns for everyone to describe their personal picture and tell about each item they chose.

The leader will restate the goals and purpose of the activity and let the participants comment about what they learned.

**Debriefing Questions/Closure:**
1. Name some of your favorite leisure activities.
2. What activities do you like to do that you don't have pictures for?
3. How do your pictures differ from everyone else's?
4. How are your pictures similar to everyone else's?
5. What do your pictures say about your leisure time?
6. What other activities would you like to learn in the next six months?

**Leadership Considerations:**
1. Some pictures may be repeated if more than one participant is involved in it.
2. The leader may ask participants to take only one picture at a time as the box keeps getting passed around.
3. The leader should make sure pictures are appropriate to the group.

**Variations:**
1. Pictures representing leisure equipment or locations (such as parks and zoos) can be used.
2. The leader may ask the participants to make up a story about the leisure activities on their collage.

**Creator:** Monika Ressel, Illinois State University, Normal, Illinois.

# Community Fun

**Space Requirements:** Classroom or activity room

**Equipment/Resource Requirements:** Paper, pencils, blackboard, chalk, phone books, newspapers

**Group Size:** Small group

**Program Goals:**
1. To increase participants' awareness of leisure and leisure activities.
2. To increase participants' awareness of community leisure resources.

**Program Description:**

**Preparation:**
The leader should have the equipment ready before the session begins. The leader may want to prepare an example or two for demonstration purposes.

**Introduction:**
The leader will introduce the activity and the goals. The leader will explain that if any questions arise, they may ask the leader at any time.

**Activity Description:**
The leader will divide the group into groups of two or three by counting off. The leader begins by discussing with the group what a leisure activity is. The leader will begin with the questions:

1. What is leisure to you?
2. What leisure activities fit into the description of leisure?
3. What activities are available in your community?
4. What leisure activities have you done in the past in your community?

The responses are written on the board for all to see. This continues until a list of 15 to 20 activities accumulates.

The leader continues the discussion with an example of where the activity might be found in the community. For example, if basketball was chosen, the activity might be done through the park district in a league or just on a driveway court.

Each group receives a phone book and a newspaper for ideas of locations. The groups are instructed to pick eight different activities that are written on the board and list the places in the community they could be found. The groups will have 10 minutes. When the time is up, the leader will ask the groups to pick a spokesperson. Each spokesperson will discuss four activities and the locations where they can be performed or found.

When all groups are finished telling the locations, each person will write two activities that he or she wants to participate in and the location and give to the leader with the pencils, newspapers and phone books.

The leader will end the discussion by using the following debriefing questions.

**Debriefing Questions/Closure:**
1. What is leisure to you?
2. What activities would you consider to be leisure?
3. What community activities were new to you?
4. Where are some good places to go to participate in leisure activities?
5. How would you get to these places?
6. What is the next place or activity you would like to try?

**Leadership Consideration:**
The leader should explain that substance-related activities should not be discussed.

**Variations:**
1. This activity could be used to discuss leisure activity benefits.

2. The activity could use home leisure resources.
3. This activity could change from listing any community leisure resource and use leisure activities that are under $5.

**Creator:** Julie Harvey, Illinois State University, Normal, Illinois.

# Leisure Treasure Hunt

**Space Requirements:** A large room with many hiding places, use of many rooms, or an outdoor area

**Equipment/Resource Requirements:** Slips of paper with instructions, envelopes, treasure

**Group Size:** Small group

**Program Goals:**
1. To improve participants' knowledge of leisure activities.
2. To improve participants' ability to use cooperative skills as a means of reaching a common goal.
3. To increase participants' communication skills with others in a group.

**Program Description:**
**Preparation:**
The leader should have slips of paper prepared and hidden ahead of time. Possible clues and hiding places include:

> Example clue:
>   This glove wasn't used by Susie in
>   cold weather.
> Answer location:
>   Softball glove.

> Example clue:
>   Round and round she goes and where
>   she stops no one knows.
> Answer location:
>   Merry-go-round.

The leader should decide on what the treasure will be and hide it.

**Introduction:**
The purpose of this activity is to provide participants with the opportunity to increase knowledge of leisure activities, increase cooperative skills and ability to demonstrate these skills, while increasing communication skills with others in a group.

**Activity Description:**
The leader will begin by stating the goals and purpose of the activity. The group should discuss types of leisure activities available to them, then hold a discussion about types of skills involved in cooperation.

The leader should give instructions for the activity. The leader should state that the participants will start off with a slip of paper that was torn out of Susie's diary. She often would tear sheets from her diary and hide them.

These slips of paper lead to clues to where she hid other diary entries about problems or feelings within her leisure lifestyle. All the clues lead to treasures that Susie discovered within her leisure life. Susie is feeling down now because she lost her first slip of paper that will lead her to the answers to her problems and the clues to find her leisure treasures.

The participants will go on a scavenger hunt.

Each participant must provide an answer to the problem on the slip of paper in order to receive the next clue to the next diary entry.

Once every participant has provided an answer to the problem, he or she may open the envelope to find the clue to the next slip of paper. Participants continue on until they receive the last clue, which tells them where the treasure is.

The leader will hold a discussion on what problems arose during the activity, what could have been done to make the activity run more effectively, and how can these skills be used in real-life situations.

The leader will restate the goals and purpose of the activity. Again, the leader will ask participants to give examples of leisure activities as well as cooperation skills.

**Debriefing Questions/Closure:**

1. What problems arose during the activity?
2. How were these problems handled?
3. How could these problems have been handled more effectively?
4. How could these skills be useful in real-life situations?
5. Why are cooperation skills so important to learn and use?

**Leadership Considerations:**

1. The leader should have the treasure located in a leisure activity room.
2. The treasure should be leisure-related items or a special activity in which to participate.
3. The leader should encourage participants to work together.
4. The leader should encourage participants to listen to each other and communicate effectively.
5. The leader should encourage participants to provide encouragement for each other.

**Variations:**

1. If there is a larger group of participants and more assistants, the activity could be made competitive by creating teams and seeing who can find the treasure first.
2. The participants could go to various areas within the facility and do a scavenger hunt, collecting various resources or answers to questions from staff and having them sign their name to their answers. The first group or individual to return would be the winner.
3. The participants can work on additional goals including knowledge of activity opportunities, problem solving, and leisure resources.

**Creator:** Renee Raczkowski, Illinois State University, Normal, Illinois.

# The Leisure Storybook

**Space Requirements:** Classroom or activity room

**Equipment/Resource Requirements:** Construction paper, magazines, markers, glue, scissors, stapler

**Group Size:** Small group

**Program Goals:**
1. To improve participants' ability to identify past, present, and future leisure involvement.
2. To improve participants' ability to recognize the importance of leisure.
3. To improve participants' ability to identify personal strengths in leisure.
4. To improve participants' self-awareness concerning a personal leisure lifestyle.

**Program Description:**
**Preparation:**
The leader should prepare booklets made of construction paper ahead of time. The leader should go through magazines and cut out activities representing leisure activities. The leader should prepare an example as a demonstration.

**Introduction:**
The purpose of this activity is to provide participants with the opportunity to explore their leisure involvement, as well as their personal strengths, while recognizing the importance of leisure in their life.

**Activity Description:**
The leader starts by stating the goals and purpose of the activity. The leader will hold a discussion about past, present, and future leisure activities.

The leader will give instructions for the activity. He or she will state that there will be three chapters to the book, the first being past, the second present, and the third future leisure involvement. The leader will show an example of a leisure storybook. The leader will instruct the participants to choose and/or draw pictures that represent their leisure involvement.

The leader should encourage participants to be creative with their books and personal strengths in leisure. The leader should give the participants 20 to 30 minutes to create their storybooks.

The leader should restate the goals of the activity. The leader should use the following debriefing questions for closure.

**Debriefing Questions/Closure:**
1. Did you learn anything new about yourself that you did not know before?
2. Are there any activities that you would add to your book?
3. Are there any activities that you no longer participate in, and why?
4. Encourage participants to share their storybook, and why they chose the pictures or words they used.
5. What activities would you like to learn in the future?
6. What is your favorite current leisure activity?

**Leadership Considerations:**
1. The leader should prepare books out of construction paper ahead of time, and look through all magazines.
2. The leader should provide an example of a leisure storybook to show the participants.
3. The leader should encourage the participants to choose or draw pictures that relate to their leisure involvement.
4. The leader should encourage the participants to be creative.
5. The leader should give participants positive reinforcement and encouragement.

**Variations:**

1. The participants may create a three-chapter storybook including physically active activities in the first chapter; activities that make use of cognitive abilities in the second chapter; and activities participated in for social purposes in the third chapter.
2. The participants may create a storybook that consists of activities that are done alone, with friends, and with family.
3. The participants may create one large book with each child contributing to one page in each chapter for any of the previously mentioned activity suggestions.

**Creator:** Renee Raczkowski, Illinois State University, Normal, Illinois.

# Mystery Match Up

**Space Requirements:** Classroom or activity room

**Equipment/Resource Requirements:** Deck of cards with pictures (two sets), corresponding question categories for participants to answer

**Group Size:** Small group

**Program Goals:**
1. To improve participants' short-term memory recall skills.
2. To improve participants' ability to articulate choices about their leisure.

**Program Description:**
**Preparation:**
The leader should prepare decks of picture cards—two cards with same picture (see examples).

**Introduction:**
The purpose of this activity is to use short-term memory recall skills and state preferences and choices about leisure.

**Activity Description:**
The leader begins by stating the goal and the purpose of the activity. The leader will explain the directions, similar to the game Concentration, and explain that each group member must wait patiently during other group members' turns. Each participant will get a turn to flip two cards, attempting to make a match. When a participant has chosen a match, he or she will have to share information about himself or herself according to the corresponding category. After all cards are gone, the participant with the most pairs wins the game.

The leader will restate the goals and purpose of the activity and let the participants comment about what they learned.

**Debriefing Questions/Closure:**
1. How easy or difficult was it to remember where the cards were?
2. What did you learn about your leisure preferences?
3. What did you learn about the leisure preferences of others in the group?

**Leadership Considerations:**
1. The leader should make sure each card has a match.
2. The leader should determine the numbers of pairs based on the abilities of group members.

**Variation:**
The activity content may be changed to reflect the needs of the participants.

**Creator:** Monika Ressel, Illinois State University, Normal, Illinois.

# Mystery Match Up

## Examples

| *Picture* | *Category* | *Questions* |
|-----------|------------|-------------|
| Tree | Place you've been | Name one leisure place you've been that you'd like to go back to. |
| Car | Place you want to go to | Name one leisure place you'd like to go to. |
| Hand | Something you're good at | Name a leisure activity that you're good at. |

# Web of Leisure

**Space Requirements:** Classroom or activity room

**Equipment/Resource Requirements:** Colored yarn or string

**Group Size:** Small group

**Program Goals:**
1. To improve participants' awareness of personal leisure interests.
2. To improve participants' awareness of leisure interests of other group members.

**Program Description:**
**Preparation:**
The leader should gather several balls of different colors of yarn or string.

**Introduction:**
The purpose of this activity is to improve participants' awareness of their own leisure interests and recognize other group members with similar leisure interests.

**Activity Description:**
The leader will state the goals and purpose of the activity. Participants each should think of at least five leisure activities they enjoy. Participants should be seated in a circle and each person gets his or her own ball of yarn. The leader will explain that each participant will get a turn to share a personal leisure interest or activity.

He or she will then ask the other group members who else has a similar leisure interest. He or she will toss the ball of yarn to every person who has a similar leisure interest, forming a web of leisure. Each activity starts a new round of web tosses.

The leader will restate the goals and purpose of the activity and let the participants comment on what they learned.

**Debriefing Questions/Closure:**
1. What are your three favorite leisure activities?
2. For each of these three activities, who else in the group also participates in them?
3. How else might you find people to participate in leisure activities?
4. How were others in the group similar or dissimilar to you?

**Leadership Considerations:**
1. The leader may have the participants pay attention to who else in the group enjoys each activity.
2. Size of yarn balls depends on how many are in each group.

**Variation:**
This format may be used for any activity where similarities and differences are important.

**Creator:** Monika Ressel, Illinois State University, Normal, Illinois.

# Silent Activity Companions

**Space Requirements:** Classroom or activity room

**Equipment/Resource Requirements:** Cards with pictures of sports activities, tape, actual equipment that coincides with pictures, large gymnasium area

**Group Size:** Small group

**Program Goals:**
1. To improve participants' use of silent communication strategies when interacting with other group members.
2. To improve participants' ability to locate leisure partners with similar leisure interests.

**Program Description:**
**Preparation:**
The leader will prepare cards (two per activity) that get taped to participants' backs and gather equipment beforehand.

**Introduction:**
The purpose of this activity is to use silent communication strategies to locate partners with similar leisure interests.

**Activity Description:**
The leader begins by stating the goals and purpose of the activity.

Before the activity begins, the pictures need to be organized so that each player will receive one. All participants need to be silent as soon as the game begins. Different activity cards will be taped to the participants' backs. They now must find their partner through hints from other group members acting out the activity that is on their back. While figuring out what's on their card, they are to help other group members by acting out the activities on their backs also.

After each participant finds his or her partner, he or she will be instructed to think of a real sports activity that he or she enjoys. Silently, that person then must find someone else within the group with the same or similar activity and take part in it; for example, partners can go to the gym area and jump rope, play basketball, or kick a soccer ball.

The leader will restate the goals and purpose of the activity and let the participants comment about what they learned.

**Debriefing Questions/Closure:**
1. How many people in the group share similar leisure interests?
2. How easy or difficult was it to identify the activities other group members were acting out.
3. How does a person go about finding people to participate with?
4. What would you do if you needed to find someone to do a leisure activity with?

**Leadership Considerations:**
1. The leader needs to take control of the activity from the beginning so that the participants will not get out of control with the acting and role-playing.
2. The leader needs to make sure that the equipment is used properly and that all group members are appropriately interacting with one another.

**Variations:**
1. Instead of acting out their interests and pursuing them, the leader could begin with a discussion of the group members' interests and see if they already know which group members have similar interests.
2. At the end of the program, a discussion could take place about different leisure activities and who would be willing to try an activity he or she is not as familiar with. Also the same program could revolve around differences, not just similarities.

**Creator:** Monika Ressel, Illinois State University, Normal, Illinois.

# What Leisure Resources Does My Community Have?

**Space Requirements:** Classroom or activity room

**Equipment/Resource Requirements:** Transportation (public or private van), maps

**Group Size:** Small group

**Program Goals:**
1. To increase participants' knowledge of leisure opportunities within the community.
2. To increase participants' knowledge of available commercial and community resources.

**Program Description:**
**Preparation:**
The leader should have the route preplanned. The leader should call facilities to set up tours, keeping in mind accessibility of facilities. The leader should pick only as many facilities as will fit into allotted time, keeping recreation interests of the participants in mind when choosing facilities.

**Introduction:**
The purpose of this activity is to improve the participants' knowledge and identification of various recreation resources available within the community.

The leader will welcome the participants and introduce himself or herself. The leader will have the participants introduce themselves and state their favorite leisure activity. The leader will explain the purpose and goals of the activity. The leader will explain where the group will be going and give the approximate time of return.

**Activity Description:**
*En route to each facility:*
The leader will discuss what the facility offers in terms of recreational programs, clubs, memberships, fees and transportation. The leader will discuss possible questions participants might ask on tour.

*At the facility:*
- The group will take the tour.
- The leader will have each participant pick up a brochure or pamphlet (if available).

*On the way back to the participants' facility:*
- The leader will discuss the facilities the group toured and ask questions such as, "What do the facilities offer?"
- The leader will have each participant tell what he or she liked or disliked about the facilities and which facility or program was of interest to him or her.
- The leader will ask each participant what he or she learned.
- The leader will discuss other commercial and community recreation facilities and ask, "What are the differences between commercial and community facilities?"

The leader will restate the goals of the field trip. The leader will encourage the participants to read brochures. Also, the leader will encourage the participants to get involved in a commercial or community recreation program.

**Debriefing Questions/Closure:**
1. Which of the facilities have you been to before?
2. Which of the facilities would you like to go back to?
3. What other facilities would you like to go to?
4. How would you get more information about these facilities?

**Leadership Considerations:**
1. The leader should be very familiar with the community and what recreation opportunities it has to offer.
2. The leader must have group control.

3. Organizational skills are necessary for preplanning.
4. This activity is intended for those participants who have adequate processing skills and are ready for community recreation involvement (e.g., necessary functional abilities and social skills to participate).

**Variation:**
Any number of resource trips may be taken depending on availability in the community.

**Creator:** Susan Osborn, Illinois State University, Normal, Illinois.

# Win, Lose or Draw Leisure Interests

**Space Requirements:** Classroom or activity room

**Equipment/Resource Requirements:** Chalkboard or dry erase board, chalk or marker, accompanying sheet for each group member, pens and pencils, stopwatch or watch with second hand, tape, blue and red pieces of paper

**Group Size:** Small group

**Program Goal:**
To improve participants' ability to identify low-cost or no-cost alternatives for leisure activities.

**Program Description:**
**Preparation:**
The leader will arrange the room so all participants can see the board. The leader will tape colored pieces of paper under chairs (the number of chairs should equal the number of participants).

**Introduction:**
The purpose of this activity is to improve participants' ability to identify low-cost leisure activities.

**Activity Description:**
The leader begins by stating the purpose and goals of the activity. The leader will discuss the idea of low-cost or no-cost leisure.

The leader will hand out the accompanying work sheet and have participants write down two low-cost and two no-cost leisure activities in which they participate currently or have participated in the past. Participants should write down sober activities. (The leader may help those having difficulty by providing clues such as, "Think of passive activities or activities you do with your family").

The participants will rip their paper apart and fold in half. The leader will pick up the papers and use them for the game (the leader will not use repeats or inappropriate activities). The leader will split the group into smaller groups or teams by having each participant look under his or her

chair for a slip of paper (red is for Group 1, blue is for Group 2). The leader will have the participants get in teams and sit in chairs near the board.

The leader will flip a coin to see who goes first. Teams will take turns drawing the ideas from the slips of paper. Each correct guess gets a point. Teams are allowed 30 seconds to respond correctly and if the team does not respond correctly, the other team can guess. In between turns the leader should briefly discuss the activity drawn and ask if anyone else participates in that activity. The leader should see how many clients think the activity is low-cost or no-cost. Is it really a no-cost activity?

The group will go through as many slips of paper as time allows. The leader will give participants a "two-minute warning." The leader will restate the goals and ask processing questions.

**Debriefing Questions/Closure:**
1. What activities did you hear today that you hadn't thought of?
2. Which of these activities could you do daily? Which of these activities could you do weekly? Which of these activities could you do monthly?
3. Which of these activities would you like to learn?

**Leadership Considerations:**
1. If participants disagree with a call, the leader is the final judge.
2. The leader should be aware of participants' limitations, and use a buddy system if a participant is unable to write or read.

**Variations:**
1. The leader should have additional no- and low-cost activities prepared ahead of time.
2. Instead of drawing activity, participants can act out the activity (charades).

**Creator:** Susan Osborn, Illinois State University, Normal, Illinois.

# Win, Lose or Draw Leisure Interests

## Low-Cost Leisure Activity

Fold 'n' Rip
– – – – – – – – – – – – – – – – – – – – – – – – – – – – – – – – – – – – – – –

## Low-Cost Leisure Activity

Fold 'n' Rip
– – – – – – – – – – – – – – – – – – – – – – – – – – – – – – – – – – – – – – –

## No-Cost Leisure Activity

Fold 'n' Rip
– – – – – – – – – – – – – – – – – – – – – – – – – – – – – – – – – – – – – – –

## No-Cost Leisure Activity

# A Day of Leisure

**Space Requirements:** Classroom or activity room

**Equipment/Resource Requirements:** Accompanying sheet, pens and pencils, brochures, newspapers, yellow pages

**Group Size:** Small group

**Program Goals:**

1. To improve participants' ability to plan and make decisions regarding leisure participation.
2. To improve participants' ability to identify a variety of recreational opportunities in the community.
3. To improve participants' ability to identify leisure opportunities within their home.

**Program Description:**

**Preparation:**

The leader will collect community resource materials and arrange the room, if necessary.

**Introduction:**

The purpose of this activity is to improve participants' decision-making skills and knowledge of home and community leisure resources.

**Activity Description:**

The leader should explain the purpose and goals of the activity. The leader will discuss types of community and home leisure resources. The leader will have the participants brainstorm aloud resources found in their home. The participants will write down ideas. (*Note:* Participants should write down only resources currently in home and/or items they would like to get in the future.) The leader should encourage participants to add to their own list, those things not mentioned aloud.

The leader should discuss community leisure opportunities. The leader will have participants write down only those resources found in their community and any additional resources not discussed.

The leader will have participants plan "a day of leisure." The participants will plan one day to spend with friends or family, and one day to spend alone. The leader will briefly show what resources are available and the participants should use these resources to plan leisure, for example, use newspaper to plan a special event or to see when a movie is playing. The leader will give the participants 10–15 minutes.

*Rules:* Participants have to fill entire day 8 A.M.–6 P.M. (or later) with leisure activities (no chores). Participants must pick at least one each of home- and community-based leisure activities.

The leader will have each participant describe one of his or her planned days (alone or with someone). If time allows the leader will have each participant describe both days.

The leader will restate the goals and ask processing questions.

**Debriefing Questions/Closure:**

1. Would this planned day be feasible? Why? Why not?
2. In what ways are your activities different alone than with others?
3. Which plan would you enjoy more after a difficult week?
4. How are your plans similar to or different from other participants?
5. How much would it cost to participate in your day?
6. Would this be a realistic day for you?

**Leadership Considerations:**

1. The leader should complete a work sheet with the group and share his or her day with the participants.
2. It is assumed participants know how to use a newspaper, phone book, and brochures to find information. If not, they need to be taught prior to this activity.

**Variation:**
Depending on the group, the leader may want to have participants list opportunities themselves and then discuss aloud.

**Creator:** Susan Osborn, Illinois State University, Normal, Illinois.

# A Day of Leisure

## Leisure opportunities in my home:

## Leisure opportunities in my community:

## A planned day of leisure with friends and/or family:

## A planned day of leisure by myself:

# Leisure Values and Attitudes Continuum

**Space Requirements:** Classroom or activity room

**Equipment/Resource Requirements:** List of Values and Attitudes Statements (for leader only)

**Group Size:** Small group

**Program Goals:**
1. To improve participants' understanding of the impact personal values and attitudes have on leisure experiences.
2. To improve participants' ability to identify personal values and attitudes related to leisure.

**Program Description:**

**Preparation:**
Note that this activity is primarily for people with substance abuse problems. The leader will arrange the room so participants have room to move about (move chairs and tables aside). The leader will review the value and attitude statements. The leader will make a copy of statements and mark the ones he or she would like to present to the group.

**Introduction:**
The purpose of this activity is to improve the participants' ability to identify and understand the impact of personal values and attitudes on leisure experiences.

**Activity Description:**
The leader begins by stating the goals and purpose of the activity. The leader will discuss the meaning of values and attitudes. The participants will brainstorm what they think is a value and an attitude. The leader will explain that people rarely think about their values and/or attitudes until someone has an opposing value or attitude. This activity will help participants to realize what their values and attitudes are and how they are differ-

ent or similar to others. The activity will also explore how others' attitudes and values affect the participants' leisure experiences.

The leader will have the participants gather in open area of the room and he or she will explain the procedures and rules of the activity.

*Rules:*
The participants will respect everyone, regardless of whether they agree or disagree with what they are saying.

*Procedures:*
- Do warmup activity to demonstrate how interaction between participants is to be done, as well as how to line up in a continuum.
- The leader will have the participants line up by age, and then by number of years at same address.
- The leader will now read a value or attitude statement, beginning with least threatening statements.
- The participants will communicate with each other to determine their place in line.
- Continuum goes from strongly agree with statement on extreme left to strongly disagree on extreme right. The center area is considered a gray area—participants may sometimes agree with the statement.
- Once participants have found their spot or grouping on the continuum they will be asked a series of questions. Not all participants will participate in questions asked for every statement read. However, it is important to get each participant to respond a minimum of two times. *Note:* The leader should get answers from each part of the continuum (extreme left and right and middle). The leader should help

discussion along by offering where he or she would stand and how the value affects his or her leisure.

*Sample Questions:*
1. Why did you choose that spot on the continuum?
2. How does your attitude or value affect your leisure?
3. Does your attitude or value hinder or help your leisure experiences?

The leader should limit discussion to a few minutes in order to present several value and attitude statements during the session. Also, the leader should note if participants are feeling uncomfortable sharing and move on to the next statement or offer his or her own thoughts. After the last statement has been read, the leader will ask processing questions.

## Debriefing Questions/Closure:
1. Which of your values and attitudes are you more aware of after completing this activity?
2. Which of your values and/or attitudes helped your leisure experiences? Which hindered your leisure experiences?
3. What statements would you add to the list?
4. How similar to or different from others in the group are you?
5. Were other people consistently in the same spot as you?

6. What does this activity tell you about your leisure?

## Leadership Considerations:
1. The leader should be aware of the mobility of all participants.
2. The leader should place himself or herself on the continuum and discuss that position for the first couple of statements to put participants at ease and to give further demonstration of how discussion is expected to progress.
3. The leader should be aware that some participants may not want to reveal personal attitudes and values—do not force participation.
4. The leader should encourage participants to be honest.
5. The leader should keep discussions on track—do not let participants stray from main point.

## Variations:
1. When leading activities with different populations and/or ages, the leader may add value and attitude statements that would be of concern to different populations and ages.
2. The leader may choose to relate all statements to leisure.

**Creator:** Susan Osborn, Illinois State University, Normal, Illinois.

# Leisure Values and Attitudes Continuum

**Time:**
1. I have too many responsibilities to have enough time for leisure activities on a daily basis.
2. I use my free time wisely.
3. "Time is money." (Benjamin Franklin)
4. "More free time means more time to waste." (Robert Hutchins)

**Motivation to Participate:**
1. Learning new things is important to me.
2. Most of my leisure activities are passive (reading, watching TV, computer games).
3. I engage in leisure activities to:
   a. meet new people.
   b. be with my friends and family.
   c. be healthier.
   d. improve myself.
4. Because of my age, I cannot do a lot of the recreation activities I use to do.
5. I am willing to try anything once.
6. Sobriety affects my enjoyment of leisure activities.
7. I exercise to relieve stress or tension.
8. Hobbies are a waste of time.
9. Park district programs are for children and/ or senior citizens.
10. I "used" to feel more comfortable in social or leisure situations.
11. I need to be the best at everything I do.
12. Lack of money keeps me from doing the leisure activities I really want to do.

**Importance of Leisure:**
1. I would rather be doing leisure activities than anything else.
2. The most important thing in life is to have fun.
3. The meaning of leisure to me is freedom of choice.

**Friendship, Family, and Intimacy:**
1. I go along with what my friends are doing, even if I do not want to.
2. I would be willing never to talk to or see my best friend again for $100,000.
3. I need a lot of love and admiration from my friends.
4. I accept and encourage intimacy in my relationships.
5. If I had $500, I would spend it on myself rather than on a family member in need.

**Justice:**
1. I am in a sporting goods store and see a person steal a pair of expensive tennis shoes. I would definitely stop the rip-off.
2. I want a world without prejudice.
3. I believe in the saying, "An eye for an eye."

**Commitment:**
1. After treatment, I plan on socializing with fellow recovering addicts.
2. I am going to make a commitment to abstinence.
3. I would make arrangements to attend 90 N.A. or A.A. meetings in 90 days.
4. I plan on arranging for substance-free recreation after treatment.

**Goal Setting:**
1. I agree with this statement, "Eat, drink and be merry, for tomorrow we may die."
2. I live for the moment.

**Self-Concept:**
1. I wish I were famous.
2. I am proud of myself.
3. I am comfortable with who I am.

# Leisure Facilities Uno

**Space Requirements:** Classroom or activity room

**Equipment/Resource Requirements:** Transportation, Uno cards, petty cash for admittance, brochures from sites not visited, folders, large envelopes

**Group Size:** Small group

**Program Goal:**
To increase participants' knowledge of community leisure resources.

**Program Description:**
**Preparation:**
The leader will arrange with sites for tours ahead of time. He or she will pick up brochures for sites that are not visited and arrange for transportation.

**Introduction:**
The purpose of this activity is to improve the participants' knowledge of community leisure resources.

**Activity Description:**
The leader should begin by stating the purpose and goals of the activity. The leader will discuss the concept of community leisure resources. Participants are given a folder that will be used as a leisure resource file.

The leader will hand out information (brochures, schedules) of places that will not be visited. These brochures are intended to help build the resource file and give participants more options for community leisure.

With each brochure, the leader will attach a Uno card, facedown, to the front. Participants will have a chance to look at cards later.

The group will travel to the sites that were prearranged (e.g., bookstore, museum, YWCA, shopping mall, skating rink, park and recreation departments, community swimming pool, theater, bowling and billiards center).

After visiting each site the leader will hand each participant an Uno card that is secured in a small envelope. The group members will talk about the facility just visited on their way to the next one.

The leader should finish up the outing at a cafe or ice cream parlor. At this time the leader will have participants look at all their Uno cards and determine who has the highest hand. Also the leader will discuss the places toured and read the brochures.

The participant that has the highest score gets choice of prizes first (all participants should get a prize).

**Debriefing Questions/Closure:**
1. What facilities were visited that you hadn't been to before?
2. Which facilities had you visited before?
3. To which facility would you need to go to participate in your favorite leisure activity?
4. To what facilities would you like to return?

**Leadership Considerations:**
1. The leader should map out route ahead of time. (Know where you are going!)
2. The leader should call ahead to make reservations for tours if needed.
3. The leader should know the area and be prepared to tell the participants about sites they may pass on the way.

**Variations:**
1. The participants may pick up cards at the site visited (staff at site will give participants envelope with name on it).

2. The group may drive by facilities they won't visit and talk about what they offer. The leader should have brochures ahead of time to hand out. This will enable the participants to see where more places are located.

**Creator:** Susan Osborn, Illinois State University, Normal, Illinois.

# Pie of Time

**Space Requirements:** Classroom or activity room

**Equipment/Resource Requirements:** Colored pencils, work sheet of pie chart, chalkboard or dry erase board, chalk or markers

**Group Size:** Small group

**Program Goals:**
1. To increase participants' awareness of appropriate times for leisure and play.
2. To increase participants' awareness of the difference between work time and free time.

**Activity Description:**

**Preparation:**
The leader will copy one work sheet for each participant, prepare one pie chart as an example, write the legend on the board, and gather other supplies.

**Introduction:**
The leader will begin the activity by discussing what leisure means to each person. The leader will ask for or provide examples of various leisure activities. Next, he or she will ask participants to identify the time of day that they usually participate in these activities.

**Activity Description:**
The leader will distribute one work sheet and set of colored pencils to each participant. The leader will explain to the participants that they will be making a day pie chart. The pie chart has 24 slices on it. Each slice represents an hour of the day. It will be their responsibility to fill in the chart according to how they spend a typical weekday.

At this point, the leader should point out the legend on the board. The leader will explain to the participants that this chart represents typical activities that they probably all do on a weekday.

When including these particular things on their own chart, they should use the appropriate colors (see the following):

- sleep (red),
- school/work (green),
- personal care (blue),
- leisure/free time (yellow), and
- other (orange).

It may be necessary to explain and give examples of personal care (bathing, grooming, eating) and other (homework, chores). It may also be helpful to write these examples on the board, next to their respective categories.

Next, the leader will explain to the participants that for each hour they spend doing the activities they should color that slice of the pie with the appropriate color. If they color it orange to represent "other," they should also write the name of the activity they are doing.

After explaining directions, the leader will instruct the participants to take a few minutes to think about what they do during the day from the time they get up to the time they go to bed. Then the participants may begin coloring their charts.

When all participants are done coloring in their pie chart the leader will have them share their charts with the group and answer the following questions (to be asked by the leader).

**Debriefing Questions/Closure:**
1. Was it easy or difficult for you to recall how you spend each hour of the day?
2. If you could change one (or two) thing(s) about how you spend your day, what would it be?
3. If there were five more hours in the day, what would you spend them doing?
4. Do you feel that you spend your time well?

**Leadership Considerations:**
1. The leader should make sure everyone in the group knows how to tell time.
2. This activity should be done during the school year. By doing it during the school year, the participants have more responsibility and time obligations and a more structured schedule, making it less demanding for memory recall.
3. Slices of pie chart should be labeled with the hours of the day.

**Variation:**
1. In addition to coloring in the slices on their pie chart, the participants can include pictures that represent each category. To do this, it may be necessary to make the pie chart on a larger piece of paper, perhaps poster board.
2. A second pie chart can be filled out describing how they spend their time on the weekend. Compare the differences and similarities.

**Creator:** Lazheta Thomas, Illinois State University, Normal, Illinois.

# Pie of Time

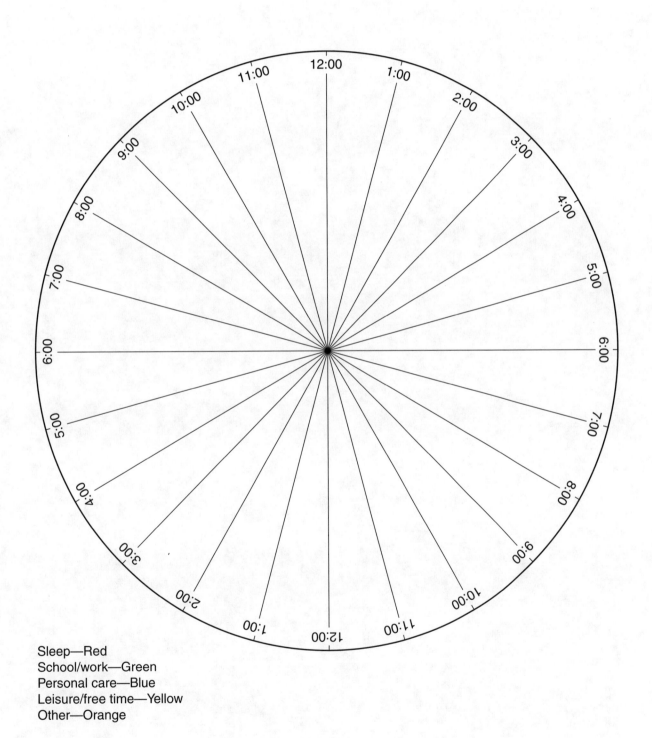

Sleep—Red
School/work—Green
Personal care—Blue
Leisure/free time—Yellow
Other—Orange

# Friendship and Social Skills

# Let's Be Friendly

**Space Requirements:** Classroom or activity room

**Equipment/Resource Requirements:** Writing utensils, accompanying form

**Group Size:** Small or large group

**Program Goals:**
1. To improve participants' ability to be friendly toward others.
2. To improve participants' ability to distinguish between appropriate and inappropriate responses to situations.

**Program Description:**
**Preparation:**
The leader should have a work sheet available for each participant and discussion topics prepared.

**Introduction:**
The leader should introduce the idea of friendliness to others. Being friendly takes practice, just like any other skill. Also, the leader should discuss appropriate times to be friendly and when people are typically approachable. The leader should emphasize highly that this is not an exercise in talking to strangers.

**Activity Description:**
Following introduction discussion, the leader will give each participant a handout (see accompanying form). He or she will have the group go through each scenario one at a time. The leader will ask the participants to respond to each of the situations with what they consider to be an appropriate act of friendliness. The leader should process their answers with regard to appropriateness, how comfortable they would feel, and how they would expect others to act in the same situation. The leader should allow ample time for discussion and differences of opinion. The leader should emphasize that while there are several responses to the scenarios, some responses are more appropriate than others.

**Debriefing Questions/Closure:**
1. In the past, how would you have responded to each of the situations?
2. What signals would tell you not to approach a person?
3. What are three other safe situations in which to use acts of friendliness?
4. What are the benefits of being friendly?
5. How would you feel if someone acted friendly toward you?

**Leadership Considerations:**
1. The leader should give examples of friendly gestures to initiate activity. He or she should have examples prepared ahead of time.
2. The leader should be prepared to point out specific safe and unsafe situations for acts of friendliness.

**Variations:**
1. The leader may change situations on the work sheet for each population group.
2. The leader may write situations on note cards and have the participants randomly pick and role-play the situations.
3. The leader may assign one week "Friendliness Week." The participants must keep records of how many times they demonstrated a friendly act.

**Creator:** Kristen Boys, Illinois State University, Normal, Illinois.

# Let's Be Friendly

How might you demonstrate friendliness in each of these situations?

1. You are standing in a long line at the grocery store and the elderly woman in front of you is short 50 cents.

2. You are walking in the hall after school and see the pitcher of your school's baseball team. The team has recently won the championship game.

3. You are at a family holiday party and notice that your cousin is just as bored as you are.

4. You call your friend whom you have known for many years. He is not home but his mom answers the phone.

5. You see your second grade teacher at the mall with her husband and two sons.

6. You are walking to the movie theater to meet your friends and notice the new boy in school standing alone outside of the theater.

# Puppet Time

**Space Requirements:** Classroom or activity room

**Equipment/Resource Requirements:** Brown lunch bag, construction paper, scissors, glue, markers or crayons, googly eyes, colorful yarn, swatches of fabric (other decorative materials)

**Group Size:** Small group

**Program Goals:**
1. To improve participants' ability to give compliments.
2. To improve participants' ability to receive compliments.

**Program Description:**
**Preparation:**
A completed example should be prepared to share with the group.

**Introduction:**
The leader should explain to the participants that they will be participating in an activity that will require them to follow directions and remain on task. The activity also will require them to give positive compliments to one another.

**Activity Description:**
The leader will begin the activity by initiating a discussion on compliments. He or she will explain to the group what compliments are and their importance. The leader will ask for and provide examples of various compliments.

Next, the leader will distribute one lunch bag to each participant. The leader will explain to the participants that they will be making a puppet out of the paper bag and the materials on the table. At this time the leader should show the example to the group. When designing the puppet, the participants should try to make it resemble themselves.

After everyone has completed his or her puppet, the leader will ask each participant to act out a role-playing situation by doing the following:

1. Introduce your puppet to the rest of the group.
2. Describe your puppet to the group.
3. Say three nice things about your puppet.
4. Give one or more compliments to other puppets in the group.

The participants should be given time both to construct puppets and discuss their attributes. The leader should make sure compliments are sincere and honest. If not, the leader should stop the activity and discuss why sincerity and honesty are important for compliments to be genuine.

The leader should close with a review on giving and receiving compliments. The following debriefing questions can be used to summarize the activity.

**Debriefing Questions/Closure:**
1. What do you like about your puppet?
2. What makes your puppet special?
3. How is your puppet different from the other puppets?
4. How easy is it to compliment someone's puppet? How difficult is it?
5. How easy is it to compliment a person? How difficult is it?
6. Name the benefits of giving honest compliments.

**Leadership Considerations:**
1. The leader should encourage participants to say different things about each puppet and not repeat what someone else has already said.
2. The leader should not rush the participants when they are trying to describe their puppet.

3. It may be necessary to assist participants with the actual making of the puppets.

**Variations:**

1. The participants could practice role-playing with their puppet before doing it in front of the group.

2. The participants could role-play how to be friendly or how to take turns with one other puppet.

3. The puppets could be used for other social skills training activities.

**Creator:** Connie Campbell, Illinois State University, Normal, Illinois.

# Puzzle Me

**Space Requirements:** Classroom or activity room

**Equipment/Resource Requirements:** Thick paper (cut out to resemble a picture frame), glue, puzzle pieces, instant camera, film

**Group Size:** Small group

**Program Goals:**
1. To improve participants' ability to give compliments.
2. To improve participants' ability to receive compliments.

**Program Description:**
**Preparation:**
The leader should instruct participants to bring in a picture of themselves or he or she should be prepared by having an instant camera on hand. The leader should gather several pieces of a jigsaw puzzle (pieces should be of a puzzle that has pieces missing, and are not of any value).

**Introduction:**
The purpose of this activity is to teach participants how to give and receive compliments. They will have the opportunity to do this throughout the activity.

At this point, it may be necessary for the leader to hold a discussion on compliments, define what they are, and give examples.

**Activity Description:**
The leader will check to make sure that everyone brought in a picture of himself or herself or the leader will take a photograph of each participant. Next, the leader will explain the directions of the activity. The leader will explain to the participants that they will be decorating a picture frame in which they will place their pictures. The frame will be decorated with puzzle pieces. When

the leader hears a person give a compliment to another individual, the leader will give that person five puzzle pieces. Participants also can give themselves a compliment to receive five more pieces of the puzzle. Last, if they are staying on task then they get five pieces for following directions. The leader should allow the group to mingle.

After each person has received approximately 25 pieces, the leader will distribute the supplies. The participants will glue puzzle pieces onto their frames. Next, they will glue the picture onto the back of the frame. The leader will conclude the activity by discussing the following questions.

**Debriefing Questions/Closure:**
1. How comfortable were you in giving compliments to someone else in the group?
2. How comfortable were you in giving compliments to yourself?
3. Name two benefits of giving compliments to others.
4. How could we remember to give compliments more often?
5. How do you feel when a compliment is a genuine one?
6. In what ways are compliments beneficial?

**Leadership Considerations:**
1. If a participant was unable to bring in a picture, the leader should have an instant camera available to use.
2. The leader must define and give examples of what a compliment is.
3. The leader should encourage and support participants when trying to compliment themselves.

4. The participants should be given enough time to think of compliments.
5. The leader should encourage participants to think of different compliments, avoid repeating what others have already said.
6. Depending on the regulations of the facility, it may be necessary to obtain permission before photographing participants.

**Variation:**
Instead of compliments, other examples of social skills, such as ways to be friendly, may be used.

**Creator:** Connie Campbell, Illinois State University, Normal, Illinois.

# Voices: Loud, Soft, Happy, and Sad

**Space Requirements:** Classroom or activity room

**Equipment/Resource Requirements:** Paper, markers, pennies, voice volume chart (see example), voice tone role-playing cards (see examples)

**Group Size:** Small group

**Program Goals:**

1. To increase participants' awareness of voice level, volume, and tone.
2. To increase participants' awareness of appropriate times to use different voice levels.
3. To increase participants' voice volume control.

**Program Description:**

**Preparation:**

The leader will have accompanying work sheets prepared for use. He or she will prepare voice tone role-playing cards with the following tones:

- afraid,
- angry,
- bored,
- demanding,
- excited,
- funny,
- gentle,
- happy,
- harsh,
- nice,
- sad,
- silly,
- soothing, and
- sorry.

**Introduction:**

This activity is designed to teach participants the importance of using their voices at the appropriate level and the appropriate times.

**Activity Description:**

The leader will begin the activity with a discussion about voice appropriateness: when it is appropriate to speak loudly, normally, or quietly. Next, the leader will explain the importance of voice tone (i.e., how it is not polite to speak to another person in a sarcastic tone when one is not happy about something).

The first part of the activity will focus on voice volume. This portion of the activity involves the voice volume chart. The participants will take turns tossing a penny onto the chart; the penny will land on either the loud, normal, or quiet portion of the chart. Each participant must think of scenarios where this volume is appropriate. The leader or participant may write each scenario in that section of the chart. When the participants have each had a few turns, the leader will give other examples and have the participants decide which volume would be appropriate. The completed chart may be used to hang on the wall as an educational poster.

The second part of the activity will focus on voice tone. The leader will give each participant a voice tone role-playing card. Each card has a specific tone of voice written on it. Each participant will role-play that tone to the group, and the group will guess what tone of voice the participant is using (e.g., Bob has a "sad" card, so Bob says the phrase of his choice in a sad tone of voice to the group). When the role-playing is completed, discuss when and where certain tones of voice should or should not be used. The leader will conclude the activity by reviewing all volume and tone scenarios and examples of appropriateness.

**Debriefing Questions/Closure:**

1. When are some times that a loud voice is appropriate? When are some times that

a quiet voice is appropriate? When are some times that a normal voice is appropriate?

2. What are some clues that let you know what volume you should use in different situations?
3. What are some consequences of using the wrong volume in different situations?
4. How does voice tone affect what we hear when someone's talking?
5. How can you make sure you're using the right volume and tone?
6. What will you practice tomorrow that you learned today?

**Leadership Considerations:**
1. The leader should give examples of situations where one would use loud, quiet, and normal voices.
2. The leader should explain what voice tone is and why it is important.

**Variation:**
Instead of having participants work as a group and take turns, the leader may give each participant a sheet of paper and have each person write down five situations that would call for loud, quiet, and normal voices.

**Creator:** Jessica Kamm, Illinois State University, Normal, Illinois.

# Voices: Loud, Soft, Happy, and Sad
## Voice Volume Chart


***LOUD***


***NORMAL***


***QUIET***

# Space Invaders

**Space Requirements:** Classroom or activity room

**Equipment/Resource Requirements:** Shoeboxes, construction paper, scissors, markers and colored pencils, glue, stencils (optional)

**Group Size:** Small group

**Program Goals:**
1. To increase participants' awareness of the importance of respecting others' personal space.
2. To increase participants' understanding of the negative aspects of having their personal space invaded.
3. To allow participants the opportunity to express creativity.

**Program Description:**

**Preparation:**
The leader will have a completed example of a decorated shoebox to share with the group.

**Introduction:**
The leader should explain to the participants that they will be doing an activity that involves recognizing the importance of personal space. At this point, define personal space as being the immediate distance surrounding one's body. The leader should explain the importance of respecting others' personal space and inform the group that when an individual's personal space is invaded, feelings of discomfort and/or uneasiness often appear.

**Activity Description:**
Following the introduction discussion, the leader will explain to the participants that they will be creating a box that will represent their "personal space." Each participant is to personalize a box to symbolize his or her personal space using con-

struction paper and markers. The leader will ask the participants to name things that they wish to keep private (e.g., favorite books, toys, secrets, body parts), that they would like to keep within their "personal space" inside the box. The leader will ask participants how they would feel if someone opened their box and "invaded their personal space" without permission. Following the discussion, the leader will restate the importance of respecting others' personal space. The leader should close with the following questions.

**Debriefing Questions/Closure:**
1. What are some appropriate ways to ask another individual to leave your personal space?
2. When are appropriate times to enter someone's personal space without asking for permission?
3. Have you invaded another individual's personal space? Was the experience pleasant or unpleasant?
4. Why is personal space and privacy important?

**Leadership Considerations:**
1. The leader should ensure that all group members have a good understanding of what *personal space* and *privacy* are before the participants begin box construction.
2. The leader should be prepared for answers or discussion from at-risk youth for whom personal space and privacy are treatment issues.

**Variation:**
The participants may act out "space invading" situations.

**Creator:** Sandra Larson, Illinois State University, Normal, Illinois.

# Faces for All Occasions

**Space Requirements:** Classroom or activity room

**Equipment/Resource Requirements:** Accompanying form, magazines to cut, glue, pencils, scissors

**Group Size:** Small group

**Program Goal:**
To increase participants' awareness of appropriate facial expressions.

**Program Description:**
**Preparation:**
The leader will copy one work sheet per participant and gather all supplies.

**Introduction:**
This activity was created to heighten participants' awareness of facial expressions.

**Activity Description:**
The leader will distribute materials to each participant and begin the activity with a discussion about body language and how a facial expression is usually as important as the words that go along with it.

Next, each participant will cut out faces from the magazines and paste them under the appropriate description, i.e., paste a happy face under the word happy.

Once faces are pasted under each heading, each participant will think of two examples that cause him or her to experience each facial expression. He or she should then write those examples above the face with the corresponding facial expression.

When all participants have completed the above steps, the group will sit in a circle. At this point, the leader will have each individual tell the group one example he or she wrote for each expression. He or she also should explain why that particular example is or is not an appropriate example for that facial expression.

The leader will conclude the activity by reviewing why certain facial expressions are more appropriate than others in certain situations.

**Debriefing Questions/Closure:**
1. What facial expressions are appropriate in the following situations:
   a. On your birthday?
   b. When your pet dies?
   c. When you do not feel good?
2. Give an example of when you knew what someone was thinking by his or her facial expression rather than what he or she said.
3. What are some benefits of sharing facial expressions?
4. Show the group your favorite facial expression.

**Leadership Consideration:**
The leader should know that the participants may misinterpret some of the facial expressions, so he or she should always have participants ask for clarification if they are confused.

**Variation:**
The participants may find a variety of facial expressions in magazines and create their own headings.

**Creator:** Jessica Kamm, Illinois State University, Normal, Illinois.

# Faces for All Occasions

Happy                                          Sad

Disappointed                                   Smiling

Confident                                      Grumpy

Angry                                          Hurt

# Character Necklace

**Space Requirements:** Classroom or activity room

**Equipment/Resource Requirements:** Leather ropes or yarn for necklaces, various colors and sizes of beads, color-coded card

**Group Size:** Small group

**Program Goals:**
1. To improve participants' ability to recognize positive characteristics of themselves that contribute to others liking them.
2. To improve participants' ability to recognize positive characteristics they wish to possess or improve upon.
3. To increase participants' awareness of their ability to control their personality characteristics.

**Program Description:**
**Preparation:**
The leader should prepare a color-coded card that shows what personality characteristic each bead color represents. He or she should separate the beads into containers, keeping like colors together and precut the necklaces to an appropriate length (14- to 22-inches). The leader should prepare a completed necklace to show to the group.

**Introduction:**
The leader should explain to the participants that they will be doing an activity that requires them to take a close look at their positive personality characteristics and those characteristics which make them likable to others.

**Activity Description:**
The leader will begin by showing the group an example of a finished beaded necklace. The leader will explain that each bead represents a personality characteristic. He or she will show the color-coded card to the participants so they are able to see which colors represent which characteristics (i.e., red is caring, blue is honesty).

Next, the leader will explain that each side of the necklace will symbolize a different thing. The right side will be positive personality characteristics the participants already possess and exercise, the left side will be positive personality characteristics they wish to acquire or improve upon.

The leader should then give each participant a special gold, silver, copper, or wooden bead to place in the center. This bead should represent *self* or who the participant is.

When the necklaces are completed, the participants will put on their necklaces with the side representing characteristics they wish to improve on over their heart. Finally, the leader will go around the room, and have each participant point out one characteristic that he or she possesses and one he or she wishes to improve on. If appropriate, the leader should hold a discussion on why it is important to recognize characteristics of one's self.

**Debriefing Questions/Closure:**
1. How difficult was it to determine what personality characteristics you have? Was it uncomfortable?
2. How will you go about trying to improve upon the characteristics you noted today? What actions will you take?
3. How do you know you need to improve upon those characteristics?
4. What characteristics are you really proud of?

**Leadership Considerations:**
1. The leader should encourage participants to be honest.
2. The leader may want to allow participants to work alone (away from others).

**Variation:**
The color of the beads may represent leisure activities, barriers, or resources.

**Creator:** Sandra Larson, Illinois State University, Normal, Illinois.

# Advertising 101

**Space Requirements:** Classroom or activity room

**Equipment/Resource Requirements:** Construction paper, scissors, old magazines, glue, markers or colored pencils

**Group Size:** Small group

**Program Goals:**
1. To improve participants' ability to recognize positive characteristics of one's self that contribute to others liking them.
2. To improve participants' ability to utilize positive self-characteristics in social settings.

**Program Description:**
**Preparation:**
The leader should have a completed product to show to the group.

**Introduction:**
The leader should explain to the participants that this activity will help them to understand the importance of knowing positive qualities of self and utilizing those qualities in various social settings.

**Activity Description:**
The leader will begin the activity by discussing what marketing and advertising are, what they do for a product, and what they can do for people. The leader should explain that each participant will create an advertising billboard. The content of the billboard will be positive, likable characteristics of one's self. The leader and participants will discuss the billboards they have seen.

Each participant will be given a large sheet of construction paper and access to the supplies.

The participants should be given approximately 45 minutes working time. Once everyone has completed his or her billboard, each participant will show and explain his or her finished "ad." The leader will emphasize activity goals and bring closure by discussing the following questions.

**Debriefing Questions/Closure:**
1. How difficult was it to determine what characteristics make you likable by others? Was it uncomfortable?
2. At any time during this activity, did you think of characteristics that you would either like to gain or improve upon? What were they?
3. What does your billboard say about you?
4. What other positive traits could you have included on your billboard?
5. How can you "advertise" your personal traits when you interact with people?

**Leadership Considerations:**
1. The leader should encourage participants to use appropriate and positive pictures to represent themselves.
2. The leader should be alert and closely watch participants to avoid off-task behaviors.

**Variations:**
1. The participants could make the billboard about a person they admire and would like to be more like.
2. The participants could bring in old pictures or other memorabilia of themselves.

**Creator:** Sandra Larson, Illinois State University, Normal, Illinois.

# Beware: Aggression Ahead

**Space Requirements:** Classroom or activity room

**Equipment/Resource Requirements:** Collage made from pictures of a variety of people cut from magazines; magazines, scissors, glue, construction paper for leader

**Group Size:** Small group

**Program Goals:**
1. To increase participants' awareness of the characteristics of an aggressive person.
2. To increase participants' ability to recognize when an aggressor is initiating an aggressive situation.

**Program Description:**
**Preparation:**
The leader should prepare a "people" collage ahead of time.

**Introduction:**
The leader should explain that the purpose of the activity is to increase awareness of the characteristics of a potential aggressor. Begin by discussing aggression and what it means.

**Activity Description:**
The leader will begin by sharing with the group the collage of different people's pictures cut from magazines. He or she will ask the group which ones appear to be aggressors and which ones do not. What are the differences? The leader should explain that all aggressors don't look alike or act alike.

The leader should ask the participants what being an aggressor means. How does an aggressor act? How does it feel when an aggressor is being aggressive towards a person?

Last, the leader will have each participant discuss ways he or she can prevent, avoid, or stop an aggressor. The leader should talk about what the participants can do if someone is being aggressive toward them or someone else.

The leader should explain that each person has the potential of being an aggressor. He or she should point out that everyone has about the same characteristics, yet everyone may not be an aggressor.

The leader should focus the participants' attention on the goals and discuss the following questions for a summary.

**Debriefing Questions/Closure:**
1. Have you ever been in a situation with an aggressive person? How did you deal with the situation or the person?
2. How can someone stop themselves from being aggressive?
3. How does it feel when you're being aggressive?
4. What are ways to get out of an aggressive situation?
5. What are alternative ways to get rid of aggressive feelings?
6. What have you learned from this session?

**Leadership Considerations:**
1. The leader should be careful not to act accusingly and label participants as aggressive.
2. The leader should be aware that aggression may be a treatment issue with some of the youth.

**Variations:**
1. All participants may work on one drawing and make up an aggressor and what they think that person would look and act like.
2. The participants, as a group, may write a short story about one person in the picture. The leader may have them explain how this person was stopped from acting aggressively toward them.

**Creator:** Sandra Larson, Illinois State University, Normal, Illinois.

# Play-Doh Personals

**Space Requirements:** Classroom or activity room

**Equipment/Resource Requirements:** One ounce of Play-Doh per person, paper bags or wax paper to protect surface of desktop, tapes and tape player

**Group Size:** Small group

**Program Goals:**
1. To increase participants' ability to recognize the importance of respecting others' personal belongings.
2. To increase participants' use of effective and polite ways to ask others for use of personal belongings.

**Program Description:**
**Preparation:**
The leader should have a completed example prepared to share with the group.

**Introduction:**
When participants enter the room, the leader should capture their attention by playing soft, calming music. The leader should introduce the purpose of the activity.

**Activity Description:**
The leader should explain to the participants that they will be doing an activity that will involve thinking about how to share their personal belongings with others and how to ask others for use of their personal belongings.

The leader will ask the participants to close their eyes and picture their favorite personal belonging. He or she should give them approximately one minute for this. After one minute, the leader will distribute one ounce of Play-Doh to each individual. Using the Play-Doh, the participants will form the object they pictured. The leader should give them about 7 to 10 minutes to complete this step.

After 10 minutes, each participant will explain what he or she formed and why he or she treasures his or her object. Then, he or she will explain how he or she would feel if that object was stolen or used by another person without permission.

After everyone has had a turn, the leader will initiate a discussion on the importance of asking permission to use other people's belongings, the consequence of using others' belongings without permission, what one should do when not given permission to use another person's belongings, and polite ways to ask others for use of their possessions.

**Debriefing Questions/Closure:**
1. Why is it important to ask others for permission to use their personal belongings?
2. Have you ever taken or used someone else's personal belongings without permission? Were there any negative consequences?
3. How would you feel if someone used or borrowed your belongings without asking?
4. What would you say to someone who used or borrowed your belongings without your permission?
5. Show us how you would ask someone to borrow his or her belonging.

**Leadership Considerations:**
1. The leader should be alert for inappropriate use of Play-Doh.
2. The leader should explain that this is not a contest to see who can get done first or who can form the most creative object.

**Variations:**
1. Cookie cutters and other supplies could be used with the Play-Doh.
2. Instead of using Play-Doh, the participants could draw their favorite personal belonging.

**Creator:** Sandra Larson, Illinois State University, Normal, Illinois.

# Thanksgiving Day Cards

**Space Requirements:** Classroom or activity room

**Equipment/Resource Requirements:** Three pieces of construction paper per participant, markers, pencils or pens, stencils (if available), Thanksgiving stickers (if available)

**Group Size:** Small group

**Program Goal:**
To improve participants' ability to express appreciation for other people.

**Program Description:**
**Preparation:**
The leader should have an example prepared to share with the group.

**Introduction:**
The leader should explain to the participants that they will be creating their own Thanksgiving Day greeting cards.

**Activity Description:**
The participants will sit at a table. The leader should inform the participants that they will be making a total of three Thanksgiving Day greeting cards. The cards are to be made for three people who they are thankful for having in their lives. The inside of the cards should contain a statement explaining the reasons why they are thankful for that person. The outside of the card can be decorated to the individual's liking. After everyone has created their cards, the participants will take turns explaining them to the group.

**Debriefing Questions/Closure:**
1. How difficult was it to choose three people to make the cards for?
2. Why is it important to let people know that you are thankful for them being in your life?
3. How do you think someone would describe the reasons they are thankful you are in their life?
4. Aside from these three individuals, who or what else are you thankful for?

**Leadership Considerations:**
1. It may be necessary to explain what it means to be thankful.
2. If the leader is unsure if individuals have three people to be thankful for, he or she may let them make fewer cards.

**Variations:**
1. This may be done another time of the year and the activity renamed accordingly.
2. Instead of cards, the group may make one large poster that describes things to be thankful for. This does not necessarily have to be specific people, but perhaps family, friends, or good health.

**Creator:** Jennifer Matkowich, Illinois State University, Normal, Illinois.

# Ways to Encourage Our Friends

**Space Requirements:** Gymnasium or large open space

**Equipment/Resource Requirements:** Note cards

**Group Size:** Small group

**Program Goal:**
To improve participants' ability to distinguish between an encouraging statement and a not so encouraging statement.

**Program Description:**
**Preparation:**
The leader should have note cards prepared with questions (see examples).

**Introduction:**
The leader should explain to the group that encouragement is an important concept to understand and practice. The idea of giving another person encouragement may lead to increasing that person's confidence level. That is something that everyone should practice. The purpose of this activity is to assist the participants in learning what an encouraging statement is and what it is not.

**Activity Description:**
The leader will begin the activity with a discussion on encouragement, explaining what it is. The leader should have the following questions on note cards and have each participant answer one question (potential answers are in parentheses):

1. Do you know what it means to be discouraged? (Feel lost, hopeless; like you try but just can't get anywhere.)
2. Can you share a time when you felt discouraged? (After a poor test performance, lost a game.)

3. Have you ever felt discouraged and did anyone say anything nice to you that really cheered you up?
4. What does encouragement mean? (The opposite of discouragement; when you say something to make another person feel better about something.)
5. Do you think that encouragement is important to give to other people, even if they are not your friends?
6. Do you think that even if the person didn't think that your encouraging words made a difference, do you think that it let him or her know that you care?

The next portion of this activity should be done in a gym or an open area. It is similar to Fetch the Bacon. The leader should have one half of the group line up on one side of the gym, the other half should line up on the other side.

The leader should number off each side so that each person has someone on the other side of the gym with the same number as himself or herself. The leader will set up the note cards on the middle line of the gym. They should be folded in half so they're standing up like a little tent.

The inner side of the note card should have statements written on them such as:

1. Alan said, "I am so stupid! I got an F on my test!" Should you say, "You are so stupid"?
2. Scott said, "I wish I could draw as well as you." Should you say, "Keep trying. It gets easier with practice"?
3. Don said, "I'm new at this school and I don't know anyone here." Should you say, "This place is pretty scary! It will take you forever to make friends"?
4. Ronny said, "I wish I could hit the ball as far as you can." Should you say, "I'm the best at baseball"?

5. Rachel said, "I can't learn anything. I got another bad grade!" Should you say, "You'll do better next time"?

6. Mark said, "None of my classmates likes me." Should you say, "We could be friends"?

7. Katy said, "Today is my first day in class. How will I make any friends!" Should you say, "You will make friends quickly. The students here are really nice"?

8. Sam said, "I wish I had more friends." Should you say, "No one likes you because you are mean and unfriendly"?

9. Ross said, "I try really hard, but I just don't understand fractions in math." Should you ask, "Would you like for me to try and help you?"

10. Bob said, "I really don't understand the questions on this work sheet." Should you say, "So what! I think this stuff is easy"?

11. Jason said, "I'm so sad that we lost our soccer game." Should you say, "Your team is really bad anyway"?

12. Joe said, "I'm no good at telling jokes like you are." Should you say, "I get my jokes from a joke book. You can borrow it if you would like to"?

The outside of the cards should have a number written on them. The leader will call out numbers that participants have been assigned. For example if the leader calls out, "Three," both threes will run to the middle of the gym and look for the note card with the number 3 written on it. The person who finds it first gets to keep it for his or her team. At this time nothing should be done with the card. The leader should instruct the person to place it on the floor, next to his or her team's line up.

The leader will proceed to call out numbers until all the note cards have been claimed by the teams. At this point the group will come back together and each person will get a card or cards claimed by his or her team. As a group, the participants will then discuss the questions on the cards.

**Debriefing Questions/Closure:**
1. The leader may ask the participants to come up with some encouraging statements to say to some of the situations on the note cards.
2. The leader may have the participants share how the encouraging comments gave the discouraged person confidence.

**Leadership Consideration:**
The leader should explain to the group that this is not meant to be a competitive activity.

**Variations:**
1. This activity could be modified to any type of game, including a board game.
2. The participants could come up with their own encouraging or discouraging situations and write those on note cards.
3. The cards could give a situation only, and the participants could create one encouraging statement and one discouraging statement.

**Creator:** Amanda L. McGowen, Illinois State University, Normal, Illinois.

# What Is a Disability?

**Space Requirements:** Classroom or activity room

**Equipment/Resource Requirements:** Accompanying work sheets, pens or pencils

**Group Size:** Small group

**Program Goals:**
1. To increase participants' knowledge and understanding of the term *disability*.
2. To increase participants' awareness of the similarities they share with other people.

**Program Description:**
**Preparation:**
The leader should have copies made of the questions for the participants.

**Introduction:**
The leader will begin the activity by discussing with the participants how they feel when they encounter a person who is different (in any way) from them. This may be a person who is of a different race, has different interests, or has a disability. The point is that the person is somehow different. After discussing how they typically feel, the leader will ask the participants how they typically act when they see someone who is different from them (e.g., stare, ask questions).

Next, the leader will ask the group the following questions. The leader should give the participants two to three minutes to brainstorm for a correct answer. After a brief discussion period of each question, the leader will state the correct answer (potential answers are in parentheses):

1. Are all the people in this room exactly alike? (No.)
2. Can you think of ways that people throughout the whole world are different? (Gender, race, physical characteristics, disabilities.)

3. What do you think of when you hear the word *disability?* (People who are deaf, blind, or mentally retarded or use a wheelchair.)
4. Can you think of any famous or local people who have disabilities? (Christopher Reeve, Helen Keller.)
5. When someone has a disability does that mean that he or she can't do anything fun or have feelings? (No, he or she can have fun and have feelings just like the rest of us.)
6. Is it important for persons with disabilities to have friends? (Yes, they have the same desire to have friends just like the rest of us.)
7. How do you feel when you see a person who has a disability in school or at a restaurant? (Awkward, may want to stare.)
8. How do you think this makes the person with the disability feel? (Some may not feel anything, they may be used to it; embarrassed, angry, hurt.)
9. Do you think it is right to call your friends names like "retard" or other names of disabilities? (No.)

**Activity Description:**
Divide the participants into pairs and give each pair a Is This a Disability? work sheet (see accompanying form). The work sheet contains a variety of possibilities. Some are true disabilities, while others are just short-term impairments or problems. The leader should have each pair work together and decide which ones are a disability. They will place a check mark next to the scenarios that they consider to be a disability. The leader should remind the participants that this is not a race so they should take their time and think through each scenario completely.

Once the participants complete the work sheet, as a group, the leader and participants will

301

go over each item and discuss why it would or would not be considered a disability. Next, the leader will ask the participants to look back at the items that are checked as being a disability and share thoughts on how people with these conditions can function well in daily activities, regardless of their disability. Some examples of how they can function include persons who use wheelchairs have ramps, drive cars; persons who are deaf can use sign language and have their vision, use special telephones; persons with visual disabilities can use guide dogs and also have their hearing.

Next, the leader will give one What Can We Do Together? scenario to each participant. (Each participant will receive one scenario from the accompanying form.) Participants will work individually to complete this portion of the activity. They will list a minimum of three things that they could do or talk about with the person in this scenario.

After the participants are finished, each will read to the group the situation he or she was given. Next, each will share with the group the three things he or she came up with. Also, each will discuss how the person in his or her scenario is similar to him or her. Last, the leader will conclude the activity by discussing that many people are different from the participants, in many ways, but overall, they have more in common with people than they have differences.

## Debriefing Questions/Closure:

1. What things have you learned that you have in common with people who have disabilities?
2. Have you ever thought about how all people are really more alike than they are different?
3. What types of daily interaction do you have with any of the types of people we talked about today? Friends or family?
4. The next time you see or meet someone with a disability, how will you react?

## Leadership Considerations:

1. The leader should allow the participants to share situations where they have been around a person with a disability. This may help to increase participants' understanding of various types of disabilities.
2. When talking about people with disabilities, the leader should use proper terminology so that the group is exposed to correct versus incorrect terminology (e.g., "people with mental retardation" rather than "the mentally retarded").

## Variations:

1. The participants may work in pairs throughout the entire activity if it seems appropriate.
2. The leader may invite guest speakers, people with disabilities, to come in and talk to the group about their disability.

**Creator:** Amanda L. McGowen, Illinois State University, Normal, Illinois.

# What Is a Disability?

## Is This a Disability?

1. Being tall.

2. Having a runny nose.

3. Being in a wheelchair.

4. Having red hair.

5. Having a hangnail.

6. Having an artificial arm.

7. Having a cut on your leg.

8. Being blind.

9. Sneezing from a cold.

10. Having a bloody nose.

12. Having a paper cut.

13. Having an upset stomach.

14. Wearing glasses.

15. Wearing a hearing aid.

16. Having a finger missing.

17. Having the flu.

18. Being overweight.

19. Being short.

20. Using a cane.

21. Having false teeth.

22. Wearing a leg brace.

23. Having a rash on your leg.

24. Using a walker.

25. Having allergies.

# What Is a Disability?

## What Can We Do Together?

Give each participant one of the following scenarios. Instruct the participants to list three things that they could do or talk about with the person described in the scenario.

1. Tommy has a patch over one eye. He likes to play soccer and football and is good at computer games.

2. Jody is from Mexico and doesn't speak any English. She has a collection of stickers and loves to eat all kinds of food.

3. Rob uses a wheelchair. He has a spinal cord injury and will never be able to walk. He loves the movie *Mulan.*

4. Justin lives in an enormous house. He goes on vacation 10 times a year and his parents own 8 cars.

5. Maria has Down Syndrome. She is in special classes at school and has a hard time speaking. She loves pizza.

6. Marcus is an American Indian. His skin is dark and his parents and grandparents know how to do native rain dances.

7. Tawanna was born with one leg shorter than the other so she uses a lift in her shoe. She likes video games and baking cookies.

8. Jose has a hearing impairment and uses a hearing aid. He collects action figures, plays Nintendo, and owns a mountain bike.

9. Barry lost the use of his right arm in a farm accident. He owns a mountain bike and collects sports cards.

10. Carla broke her leg on the playground. She uses crutches and can't walk very fast.

# Trust Circle

**Space Requirements:** Classroom or activity room

**Equipment/Resource Requirements:** None needed

**Group Size:** Small group

**Program Goals:**
1. To increase participants' comfort level with trusting someone else.
2. To increase participants' ability to identify reasons to trust or mistrust someone.

**Program Description:**
**Preparation:**
No special preparation needed.

**Introduction:**
The leader will begin the activity by initiating a discussion about trust. He or she will ask the participants what trust is and how they define it. The leader may ask for and use examples as needed. Next, he or she will ask the participants the following questions:

1. How long does it take to trust someone?
2. How long does it take to lose someone's trust?
3. What specific behaviors must one take in order to establish a trusting relationship?

**Activity Description:**
The leader will divide the group into groups of three. The leader should explain to the group that each participant will have the opportunity to fall backward into another person's hands and arms. Each person also will have the opportunity to catch someone.

The leader should establish ground rules. If the participants are unable to hold the person up then they can gently let him or her down to the floor. The leader should give the group a few minutes to make up additional ground rules and/or behaviors that will not be tolerated, i.e., no pushing, no fooling around, and to remain on task.

When the groups have chosen who will do which task first, instruct one participant in each trio to fall backward. The second person is to catch the person and then gently push him or her back to the standing position. The third person is to stand next to the catcher if help is needed to reposition the participant. If the third person is nervous, the leader or a staff member will be a spotter. After each person in the trio has gone once, the activity will be repeated with the person who is falling closing his or her eyes (only if the person falling backward feels comfortable).

**Debriefing Questions/Closure:**
1. How did you feel when you were being caught? How did you feel when you were catching? How did you feel when you were spotting?
2. How well did you trust your group members?
3. What did group members do to reinforce feelings and thoughts of trust?
4. Did group members do anything to generate feelings of mistrust?
5. What are things we can do in our lives to generate feelings and thoughts of trust in others?
6. What have you done in your lives that generated trust or mistrust?
7. What characteristics help us trust someone?
8. What can you do better to help people trust you?

**Leadership Consideration:**
The leader should keep an eye on each group to make sure that everyone is paying attention to the person who is falling backward.

**Variations:**

1. Instead of falling backward, the group can use blindfolds and lead each team member through a large (unfamiliar) area.

2. The group could also blindfold participants and give them directions to follow from there.

**Creator:** Lazheta Thomas, Illinois State University, Normal, Illinois.

# Expressing Opinions

**Space Requirements:** Classroom or activity room

**Equipment/Resource Requirements:** Writing utensils, accompanying form

**Group Size:** Small group

**Program Goals:**
1. To increase participants' ability to openly express their thoughts and opinions to peers.
2. To increase participants' ability to accept others' thoughts and opinions without criticism.

**Program Description:**
**Preparation:**
The leader should make one copy of the work sheet for each participant. The leader should choose a theme to discuss; the example here is "favorite movie."

**Introduction:**
The leader should explain to the participants that they will be doing an activity that will give them the opportunity to tell others about their favorite movie. They also will learn about the others' favorite movies.

The leader should set the ground rules. It will be important to listen to the reasons why each person chooses a particular movie as his or her favorite. If participants do not hold the same opinion, they are not allowed to say negative comments. It is important to respect others' opinions.

**Activity Description:**
The participants will form a circle (either by sitting on the floor or in chairs). The leader will distribute one pencil and work sheet to each person. As a group, the leader and participants will read over the work sheet. Next, the leader will give the group 10–15 minutes to individually complete the work sheet.

Once everyone has completed the questions, each person will read his or her answers to the group, explaining the reasons why he or she chose the movie he or she did. The leader should encourage the group to discuss the differences and similarities between the answers and opinions. The leader will conclude the activity by discussing the following questions.

**Debriefing Questions/Closure:**
1. Why is it important to use good listening skills while others are talking?
2. Why is it important to always respect others' opinions?
3. If you disagree with a person about something, how can you positively say that you hold a different opinion?
4. How do you show someone you respect his or her opinion?

**Leadership Consideration:**
The leader should be alert to participants' reactions to others' comments. Help may be needed to frame commands positively.

**Variations:**
1. The participants may choose a topic they would like to discuss.
2. Instead of filling out the work sheet by themselves, each person could act as a reporter and interview another person in the group.
3. Instead of having a work sheet to fill out, the group can have open discussion on the topic chosen.

**Creator:** Lazheta Thomas, Illinois State University, Normal, Illinois.

# Expressing Opinions

## Example Work Sheet Based on Movies

Choose a movie that you have always had an interest in or that you consider to be your favorite movie. Take a few minutes to think about this movie. Be prepared to explain the movie in great detail.

    Please answer the following questions as completely and with as much detail as possible:

1. What is your favorite movie?


2. Who were your favorite characters? Why?


3. What was the movie about? Explain.


4. Explain your favorite scene, and why it is your favorite.


5. Why is this your favorite movie?


6. Where did you see this movie?


7. Whom did you go with to see the movie?

# Social Tag

**Space Requirements:** Outdoor area or gymnasium

**Equipment/Resource Requirements:** None

**Group Size:** Small group

**Program Goals:**
1. To increase participants' knowledge on introduction techniques.
2. To increase participants' knowledge of appropriate conversational topics.

**Program Description:**
**Preparation:**
The leader should make sure the running area is open and safe.

**Introduction:**
The purpose of this activity is to allow the participants to exercise appropriate introduction techniques and to increase participants' ability to work with peers in a cooperative and competitive environment.

**Activity Description:**
The leader will begin the activity by discussing social skills. The participants will be asked to give examples of the way in which they introduce themselves to other people. The group then will discuss the most appropriate introduction techniques to use. The participant also will discuss appropriate conversation topics to discuss with the person to whom one is being introduced.

Following the discussion, the activity will begin. The leader will ask for volunteers or assign two people to be the Social Taggers. If a participant is tagged then he or she must stay in the frozen position until someone comes to unfreeze him or her.

A person who is tagged must properly exercise introduction techniques to the person who is untagging. This is done by shaking the person's hand and introducing himself or herself.

Once everyone has been tagged or after 5–10 minutes, two new people will be chosen to be the Social Taggers and the second round will be played. During this second round, not only will individuals who have been tagged have to properly introduce themselves, but they also will have to say to the person untagging them one thing that they like to do and ask that person for one thing he or she likes to do, for example, "I like to play softball. What sports do you like?"

The participants will sit in a circle and refocus on the goals of appropriate introduction techniques and conversational topics. The leader should use the following debriefing questions.

**Debriefing Questions/Closure:**
1. Give an example of how you would introduce yourself to someone new.
2. What would be five topics appropriate for starting a conversation with someone new?
3. Give a situation where it would not be appropriate to introduce yourself to someone.
4. What topics would be inappropriate for conversations with people you have just met?

**Leadership Considerations:**
1. The leader should demonstrate how to properly use introduction techniques.
2. The leader should make sure everyone understands the rules about how to untag someone.
3. The leader should demonstrate how to tag so that no one gets hurt (e.g., no pushing).

**Variations:**
1. The leader may vary the ways in which one becomes untagged.
2. The leader may have only one person be the Social Tagger.

**Creator:** Connie Campbell, Illinois State University, Normal, Illinois.

# Social Skills Trivia

**Space Requirements:** Gymnasium, large classroom, large activity room, or an open field outside with a large running area

**Equipment/Resource Requirements:** Accompanying form, 44 index cards, list of trivia questions, two noisemakers (e.g., whistle, bell), one die, chalkboard or notepad to keep score on, stopwatch or 30 second timer, prizes for each team (e.g., candy, gum)

**Group Size:** Small group of an even number of participants

**Program Goals:**
1. To improve participants' ability to work co-operatively with peers.
2. To increase participants' ability to follow directions.
3. To increase participants' awareness of proper social skills.

**Program Description:**
**Preparation:**
The leader should prepare all note cards and trivia questions prior to the start of the game. Four of the note cards should identify each of the four categories. The trivia questions should be written on the remaining note cards.

**Introduction:**
The purpose of this activity is to encourage participants to work cooperatively while participating in a competitive game which requires knowledge regarding appropriate social skills.

**Activity Description:**
The leader will inform the participants that they will be participating in an activity which will challenge their knowledge of appropriate social skills. At this point it may be necessary for the leader to explain and give examples of what appropriate social skills are.

The leader will divide the group into two equal teams. The leader should explain the rules of the game to the groups. The rules are as follows:

1. Each team will be given a noisemaker.
2. Both teams will roll the die to determine which team will go first. The team with the highest roll will go first.
3. There will be 4 categories and 10 questions under each category.
4. The team going first will choose the category from which the question will come.
5. The leader will read the questions. After the question has been read completely, the first team to "noise in" will be given the opportunity to respond:
   a. If the team responds correctly, the team will receive 1 point and will choose the next category.
   b. If the team responds incorrectly, the opposing team will be given a chance to respond.
   c. If the opposing team responds correctly, they will not receive a point, but rather, will be able to choose the next category.
   d. If no team responds correctly, the initial team to respond will choose the next category.
6. Teams must reach a mutual agreement on the answer before it will be accepted.
7. Teams will be given 30 seconds, following the "noise in," to respond.

Once the rules have been explained, the leader will distribute noisemakers and begin play. Play will end when all questions have been answered or until session time runs out. The leader will end the activity by discussing the following questions.

**Debriefing Questions/Closure:**

1. What questions did you have difficulty answering?
2. Which of the social skills, identified in the trivia questions, do you use daily? Identify any social skills which you could work toward improving.
3. What, if anything, was difficult about working cooperatively with your peers?
4. In what ways did your team work cooperatively? How did cooperation increase your success while playing this game?

**Leadership Considerations:**

1. The leader may want another individual to act as the judge to determine which team "noises in" first.
2. The leader should make sure each team member receives a prize by the end of the game.
3. The leader should remind the group that this is a somewhat competitive activity, but the most important thing to remember is to work together to answer the questions correctly.
4. The leader should encourage all individuals to participate.

**Variation:**

The trivia game could be related to leisure resources, leisure activities, or diversity among cultures.

**Creator:** Theresa M. Connolly, CTRS, Illinois State University, Normal, Illinois.

# Social Skills Trivia

## Communication Skills

1. True or false: Acting out or speaking inappropriately may be seen as negative attention seeking.
   (*True*)
2. True or false: A roadblock to communication might be ignoring distractions.
   (*False*)
3. True or false: When trying to communicate to another individual, it is appropriate to get angry if the person does not understand you the first time you send your message.
   (*False*)
4. True or false: It is important, when communicating with others to use language or words that others are able to understand.
   (*True*)
5. True or false: It is impossible to communicate with someone who may be hearing or visually impaired (deaf or blind).
   (*False*)
6. When giving directions, you should:
   a. only have to give the directions once.
   b. be willing to reexplain the directions if they are not understood.
   c. become angry with those individuals who do not understand your directions.
   d. All of the above are appropriate.
   (*B*)
7. When trying to get someone's attention who is talking to another person, you should:
   a. wait until the person is done speaking and then say his or her name to gain his or her attention.
   b. shout his or her name until he or she acknowledges you.
   c. tug on the person's clothing until he or she turns your way.
   d. None of the above are appropriate.
   (*A*)

8. True or false: Distractions which might interfere with communication could include the television, the radio, and/or other conversations.
   (*True*)
9. True or false: If someone is trying to communicate with you it is appropriate to respond by not looking at the person.
   (*False*)
10. Someone might think you were closed to communication if you:
    a. sat forward and smiled.
    b. participated in the conversation.
    c. sat with your arms and legs crossed and rolled your eyes constantly.
    d. None of the above indicate being closed to communication.
    (*C*)

## Respecting Others

1. True or false: When discussing the answer to a question, you should always argue and say your answer is correct, regardless of what the correct answer may be.
   (*False*)
2. True or false: It is appropriate to steal someone's belongings if the owner leaves them out rather than puts them away.
   (*False*)
3. An example of calling someone a name may include:
   a. saying nothing rather than saying something mean.
   b. calling someone "stupid."
   c. calling the person by his or her first name.
   d. None of the above.
   (*B*)
4. True or false: Destroying someone's personal property is not an appropriate way to display anger.
   (*True*)

5. True or false: It is OK to make fun of some-one, as long as he or she deserves it.
(*False*)

6. True or false: Teasing others is not polite and may hurt someone's feelings.
(*True*)

7. When staff asks you if you have behaved in-appropriately, you should:
   a. lie to get out of trouble.
   b. blame someone else for your behaviors.
   c. take responsibility for your behaviors.
   d. None of the above are correct.
(*C*)

8. True or false: When someone has upset you, it is OK to go to your friends and talk badly about the person behind his or her back.
(*False*)

9. True or false: Rolling your eyes is an appro-priate way to let someone know that you are not interested in what he or she has to say.
(*False*)

10. When another person has hurt your feelings, or done something you dislike, you should:
   a. yell at and hit that person.
   b. explain to the person that you disagree or that their actions have made you feel uncomfortable.
   c. get your friends and gang-up on the per-son.
   d. All of the above are acceptable.
(*B*)

# Social Skills in the Kitchen

1. True or false: Belching after a meal is a com-pliment to the chef and should be done aloud at the dinner table.
(*False*)

2. When eating dinner, your napkin should be placed where?
   a. On the table.
   b. On your lap.
   c. Tucked into the neck of your shirt.
   d. None of the above.
(*B*)

3. True or false: You should cover your mouth when you sneeze, especially around food and other people.
(*True*)

4. After you finish eating your meal, you should:
   a. get up and leave the table.
   b. play with your food until the rest of the group is done eating.
   c. ask to be excused and take your plate into the kitchen.
   d. All of the above are acceptable.
(*C*)

5. True or false: There is no need to wash your hands before you handle food.
(*False*)

6. While eating your meal, you decide you would like some salt and pepper, you should:
   a. reach across the table and grab the shak-ers yourself.
   b. shout at the person across the table to give you the salt and pepper.
   c. politely ask your neighbor to please pass the salt and pepper.
   d. None of the above are appropriate.
(*C*)

7. True or false: It is acceptable to eat any meal using your fingers.
(*False*)

8. True or false: It is considered polite and proper to slurp while eating your soup.
(*False*)

9. True or false: When washing the dishes, it is important to use both soap and water.
(*True*)

10. True or false: When you get up from the table, you should leave your chair out so it is ready for the next person to sit in it.
(*False*)

# Compliments All Around

**Space Requirements:** Classroom or activity room

**Equipment/Resource Requirements:** One piece of paper per participant, writing utensils

**Group Size:** Small group

**Program Goals:**
1. To improve participants' ability to give compliments.
2. To improve participants' ability to receive compliments.

**Program Description:**
**Preparation:**
The leader should prepare an example to share with the group.

**Introduction:**
The leader should explain to the participants that they will be doing an activity that requires them to give each other compliments.

**Activity Description:**
The participants will sit at a table. The leader should explain the directions of the activity. To begin, each participant will receive a blank piece of paper and a writing utensil. The participants will end up passing around and sharing this piece of paper with the entire group. They are to write their name on the top of the paper. Next, they should number the paper (going down) on the left-hand side. The amount of numbers should equal the total number of individuals in the group. The leader should discuss a few rules to writing compliments about group members. Compliments should be honest, true, and genuine. Compliments are to help allow a person to feel better, not to be hurt. The group may develop more guidelines as necessary.

Once these steps are completed the participants are to pass their paper to the left. Each time a person receives another individual's paper he or she is to write a positive thing about that person. The statements can be thoughts or complete sentences. They can be physical or personality characteristics; for example, a good friend, a fun person, a pleasant smile, a nice laugh, or anything related. Once everyone in the group receives his or her paper back, each individual should read his or her paper to the group.

The leader should focus the group members on improving their skills in giving and receiving compliments and end the session with the following questions.

**Debriefing Questions/Closure:**
1. How difficult was it to state only one positive characteristic about each group member? What else would you have said if you could give unlimited compliments?
2. What were you most surprised about on your own sheet of paper?
3. How does it feel to give more compliments?
4. What could you do to give more compliments to other people?
5. What could you do to get more compliments from other people?

**Leadership Considerations:**
1. The leader should decide beforehand if the participants should write their names next to the positive statement.
2. In order for this activity to be successful, the group needs to know each other fairly well.

**Variation:**
Instead of passing the sheets of paper around to each group member, each participant may write positive characteristics about each person on his or her own paper and then have the group try and guess who he or she is describing.

**Creator:** Jennifer Matkowich, Illinois State University, Normal, Illinois.

# Clay and Me

**Space Requirements:** Classroom or activity room

**Equipment/Resource Requirements:** Clay or clay substance and blindfolds

**Group Size:** Small group

**Program Goals:**
1. To increase participants' understanding of a situation without the ability of sight.
2. To increase participants' awareness and personal attitudes toward people with disabilities.

**Program Description:**
**Preparation:**
The leader should gather clay and blindfolds.

**Introduction:**
This activity is used to create awareness of people with visual impairments. This experience will allow people with normal vision to experience what it might be like to be a person with a visual impairment. The activity intent is not to discourage people but to increase their understanding of people with visual impairments.

**Activity Description:**
The leader should have the participants sit at desks or tables. The participants should then put a blindfold on. The leader will instruct the participants that this activity will not have the full effect if the blindfold is not correctly applied. The leader will then give each participant one piece of clay. The leader then tells the participants to form the clay into an object that is used for recreation or a form of leisure. After about 20 minutes, or as long as time allows, the participants then will put the clay down and remove their blindfolds. The participants then will discuss what they felt while creating the object and why they created the object.

The leader will collect the clay after the discussion. The activity was developed to assist participants in understanding what it feels like to be an individual with a visual impairment. At the same time, the participants expressed what they enjoyed as leisure activities. This activity can bring out a lot of feelings toward people with visual impairments and how it feels.

Debriefing questions follow that can be used for summary discussion.

**Debriefing Questions/Closure:**
1. How did you feel while you were molding your clay?
2. What do you think it would be like to have a visual impairment?
3. What are some devices or techniques used by people with visual impairments in their daily lives?
4. What kind of training would you need to work these devices or use these techniques?

**Leadership Consideration:**
The leader should consider the cognitive ability of the participants.

**Variations:**
1. Participants could create their face or an animal.
2. Participants could work together to form a scene, such as farm, school playground, or zoo.

**Creator:** Julie Harvey, Illinois State University, Normal, Illinois.

# Circle of Friendship

**Space Requirements:** Classroom or activity room

**Equipment/Resource Requirements:** Plastic rope, beads, containers

**Group Size:** Small group

**Program Goals:**

1. To increase participants' knowledge of personal friendship qualities.
2. To increase participants' ability to identify friendship qualities of other individuals.
3. To increase participants' ability to verbally state positive friendship qualities to others within a small group.

**Program Description:**

**Preparation:**

The leader should have plastic rope cut in 18- to 22-inch lengths ahead of time. Also, the leader should have beads placed in individual containers. About five beads per participant should be placed in each container (if there are 10 participants, then 50 beads should be placed in each container).

**Introduction:**

The purpose of this activity is to provide participants with the opportunity to increase knowledge of friendship qualities; identifying one's own qualities and other individuals' qualities, while allowing participants to verbally state positive friendship qualities to another individual.

**Activity Description:**

The leader starts by stating the goals and purpose of the activity. He or she will ask the participants to discuss what positive friendship qualities are.

The participants will sit in a circle. The leader will give instructions for the activity, pass out the plastic rope and beads to the clients, and choose an individual to begin the activity by sitting in the center of the circle.

One at a time, each person on the outside of the circle must state a positive friendship quality about the individual in the center of the circle.

After the participant states a positive friendship quality to the individual in the center, he or she must give the person in the center a bead to place on his or her plastic rope for his or her bracelet or key chain.

The participant on the outside of the circle may state as many qualities as he or she would like. However, the participant in the center will receive one bead for every quality stated by the person on the outside of the circle. The participants continue to take turns in the center until they have a complete bracelet or key chain.

The leader should hold a discussion about what the participant learned about his or her friendship qualities, and what qualities the participants look for in others. The leader should restate the goals and purpose of the activity and close with the following summary questions.

**Debriefing Questions/Closure:**

1. What qualities make a good friend?
2. What qualities do you have that make you a good friend?
3. What friendship qualities do you look for in others?
4. What qualities do your friends have that make them a good friend?
5. What qualities can you work on to become a better friend?

**Leadership Considerations:**

1. The leader should demonstrate the activity. He or she should have a completed friendship bracelet or key chain to show.

2. The leader should assist participants with helpful suggestions, if necessary.
3. The leader should allow participants to pass if they want to.
4. Participants should be familiar with each other.

**Variation:**
The activity could be used to evoke positive statements about other participants in the group.

**Creator:** Renee Raczkowski, Illinois State University, Normal, Illinois.

# Social Charades

**Space Requirements:** Classroom or activity room

**Equipment/Resource Requirements:** Social skills topic cards and bonus cards

**Group Size:** Small group

**Program Goals:**

1. To improve participants' ability to identify appropriate social interactions in everyday situations.
2. To improve participants' ability to identify cooperative skills in everyday situations.

**Program Description:**

**Preparation:**

The leader should have poster board precut into squares and supplies ready. He or she should prepare social skills topic cards and bonus cards. Examples of social skills topics cards include:

- Ask a friend to go to the mall with you.
- Ask a friend to do you a favor.
- Introduce yourself to a stranger.

**Introduction:**

The purpose of this activity is to provide the participants with an opportunity to demonstrate knowledge and skills of appropriate social interaction and cooperation in order to participate successfully within the small group activity.

**Activity Description:**

The leader will state the goals and purpose of the activity. He or she should involve the participants in a discussion about appropriate social interactions and cooperative actions, and how they are used in different situations.

The leader will give instructions for the activity. He or she will state that each participant will pick a partner and act out, in front of the group, a topic on the card. He or she will state

that the first person to guess will be next to choose a partner, and act out a topic.

The leader should demonstrate the activity. He or she will tell participants that they will be given a bonus card each time they demonstrate appropriate social skills. If the participant earns at least five bonus cards, he or she will receive a prize.

The leader should restate the goals and purpose of the activity. Debriefing questions follow.

**Debriefing Questions/Closure:**

1. What social skills were discussed?
2. What appropriate social interactions did you demonstrate?
3. What was the result of your actions?
4. What social skills do you need to improve?
5. Why are social skills important to learn and use?
6. How does one learn social skills?

**Leadership Considerations:**

1. The leader should encourage participants to practice appropriate social skills discussed previously.
2. The leader should remind each participant that everyone has a chance to be a winner.

**Variations:**

1. When working in a larger group, the leader may choose to do the activity as team charades. The leader will form groups of three or more and have the participants act out an activity together.
2. The participants could choose ideas to act out in front of the group.
3. This activity may be used to learn about leisure resources. Participants can act out different leisure resources.

**Creator:** Renee Raczkowski, Illinois State University, Normal, Illinois.

# Animal Compliments

**Space Requirements:** Classroom or activity room

**Equipment/Resource Requirements:** Animal crackers and napkins

**Group Size:** Small group

**Program Goals:**
1. To increase participants' ability to give compliments to another person.
2. To increase participants' ability to receive compliments from peers.

**Program Description:**
**Preparation:**
The leader should have animal crackers and napkins for the activity.

**Introduction:**
The purpose of this activity is to increase participants' ability to give and receive compliments.

**Activity Description:**
The leader starts by stating the goals and purpose of the activity. He or she will hold a discussion about compliments and talk about how genuine compliments are meaningful to people.

The leader will pass the bag of animal crackers around and state that the participants should take as many as they might need, but no more than 10. The leader should instruct the participants to choose a partner. After they have chosen their animal crackers and a partner, they will state positive comments directed to their partner, for each animal cracker they have. They will give their animal crackers to their partners as they give them a compliment. Once both partners have exchanged comments, they may eat their animal crackers.

The leader will hold a discussion on the importance of compliments and situations where compliments would be appreciated.

The leader should restate the goals and purpose of the activity. The following debriefing questions may be used for closure.

**Debriefing Questions/Closure:**
1. What is a compliment?
2. What is the difference between a genuine compliment and a fake one?
3. When should you give compliments to people?
4. What are good ways to respond to compliments?
5. Why are compliments important?

**Leadership Considerations:**
1. The leader should suggest that the participants might want to think before they decide to take 10 animal crackers.
2. If an animal cracker is eaten before a participant's turn, the participant will have to make an additional positive comment per animal cracker eaten.
3. The leader should encourage participants to give positive and not negative comments.
4. The leader should assist participants when they have difficulty with ideas.
5. Participants should know one another reasonably well.

**Variations:**
1. This may be used as an icebreaker. The participants should state as many things about themselves according to how many animal crackers they choose.
2. The participants could name as many resources or activities as they have animal crackers.

**Creator:** Renee Raczkowski, Illinois State University, Normal, Illinois.

# The Proper Picnic

**Space Requirements:** Classroom or activity room

**Equipment/Resource Requirements:** Tablecloth, silverware, plates, finger food, situation cards

**Group Size:** Small group

**Program Goals:**
1. To improve participants' ability to use appropriate table manners.
2. To improve participants' ability to use appropriate language at the table.

**Program Description:**
**Preparation:**
The leader will gather all supplies and prepare the situation cards. Possible situations include:

- Show us how you ask for the salt and pepper to be passed to you.
- Show us how to eat with your mouth closed.
- Start a conversation with the person to your right.

**Introduction:**
The purpose of this activity is to provide participants with the opportunity to display appropriate personal table manners both within a mock setting and within daily life.

**Activity Description:**
The leader begins by stating the goals and the purpose of the activity. The leader should explain appropriate manners and give participants the opportunity to read situation cards and demonstrate appropriately the action described on the card. The leader should give the participants the opportunity to take turns setting the table and asking for and receiving food. The leader should discuss the importance of appropriate conversational topics. The leader should distribute materials and assist participants in making appropriate decisions and practicing table manners.

The leader should restate the goals and purpose of the activity and let the participants comment about what they learned. Using the following debriefing questions will help reinforce the goals and purpose.

**Debriefing Questions/Closure:**
1. Demonstrate the right way to ask for food to be passed to you.
2. Demonstrate where to place your napkin while you're eating.
3. Name two topics appropriate for table conversation.
4. When are good table manners appropriate?

**Leadership Considerations:**
1. The leader should make sure to reward appropriate behavior.
2. The leader may need to demonstrate manners and have participants then perform.

**Variation:**
Make the setting more formal to mimic a formal restaurant.

**Creator:** Monika Ressel, Illinois State University, Normal, Illinois.

# Getting to Know About Friendship

**Space Requirements:** Classroom or activity room

**Equipment/Resource Requirements:** Cutout paper circles, large Popsicle sticks, crayons and markers, table to resemble puppet theater, words that represent good and bad friendship

**Group Size:** Small group

**Program Goals:**
1. To improve participants' ability to distinguish between being a good and bad friend.
2. To improve participants' ability to portray characteristics of being a good friend.

**Program Description:**
**Preparation:**
The leader will gather supplies, create a sample puppet, create theater or backdrop, and create a list of words that participants can relate to. Possible good friendship words include:

- loyal,
- trustful,
- helpful,
- good listener, and
- respectful of property.

Possible bad friendship words include:

- hurtful,
- lying,
- disrespectful,
- tells secrets, and
- destructive.

**Introduction:**
The purpose of this activity is to provide the participants with an opportunity to engage in a social interaction role-play experience and explore the idea of what friendship means.

**Activity Description:**
The leader starts by stating the goals and purpose of the activity. He or she will ask the participants to identify characteristics of a good friend and a person who isn't a good friend. The leader will distribute circles and instruct the participants to create two pictures of friendship, good and bad, one on each side of the circles. They will glue the circles onto the Popsicle sticks to create puppet-like figures.

The leader will distribute the words and the participants will be asked to role-play a situation that involves the words. Role-playing can take place either with partners or alone.

The leader should restate the goals and the purpose of the activity and let the group comment about what they learned or their reactions.

**Debriefing Questions/Closure:**
1. What are characteristics of a good friend?
2. What characteristics show that a person is not a good friend?
3. Are you usually a good friend or not, to people you know?
4. What could you do to be a better friend to people you know?
5. What will you work on, to be a better friend?

**Leadership Considerations:**
1. The leader should tailor the words to the needs of the group.
2. The leader should have a puppet completed to show the group.

**Variation:**
Ask participants to write a play about friendship and act it out.

**Creator:** Monika Ressel, Illinois State University, Normal, Illinois.

# The Jellybean Jamboree

**Space Requirements:** Classroom or activity room

**Equipment/Resource Requirements:** Jellybean candy, plastic eggs

**Group Size:** Small group

**Program Goals:**
1. To improve participants' ability to give compliments to peers.
2. To improve participants' ability to receive compliments from peers.

**Program Description:**
**Preparation:**
The leader will purchase jellybean candy and plastic eggs. The leader will refer to the color-coded chart and put a number of jellybeans in each plastic egg.

**Introduction:**
The purpose of this activity is to provide participants with the opportunity to give and receive compliments from peers.

**Activity Description:**
The leader begins by stating the goals and the purpose of the activity. He or she will instruct the participants of the directions and explain that each group member must wait patiently while the other group members are going. Each participant will receive an egg with different color jellybeans in them. The different colors will represent many characteristics of a friend. The participants will take turns, and for every bean they must say something nice about another peer according to the color. For example, as the compliment giver hands a white jellybean to a person, he or she says, "I think you are a good listener because you followed directions to this activity."

As the compliment is given, the person saying the compliment gives the jellybean to the compliment receiver. The compliment recipient should give an appropriate response. Jellybeans are only to be eaten after all compliments are given.

After all jellybeans are distributed (and traded for flavors if necessary) and eaten, the participants will be allowed to comment on the ways that their peers complimented them.

The leader should restate the goals and purpose of the activity and let the participants comment about what they learned.

**Debriefing Questions/Closure:**
1. What is a compliment?
2. How do you feel when you give a compliment?
3. How do you feel when you receive a compliment?
4. Why is it important to compliment others?
5. In what ways are compliments important to us?
6. What can you do to remember to give more compliments?

**Leadership Considerations:**
1. The leader may need to start by stating rules, such as all compliments must be genuine.
2. The leader should be able to give an example for each participant.
3. The participants need to know each other reasonably well.

**Variation:**
The participants may determine the meaning of the different colors.

**Creator:** Monika Ressel, Illinois State University, Normal, Illinois.

# The Jellybean Jamboree

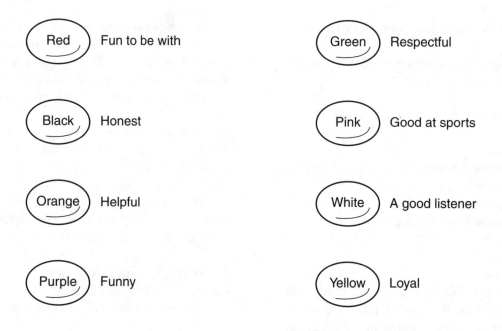

Red — Fun to be with

Green — Respectful

Black — Honest

Pink — Good at sports

Orange — Helpful

White — A good listener

Purple — Funny

Yellow — Loyal

Example: I think you are _____ because. . . .

# I Can Use Appropriate Language

**Space Requirements:** Classroom or activity room

**Equipment/Resource Requirements:** Prerecorded tape, tape player, accompanying form, pencils

**Group Size:** Small group

**Program Goals:**
1. To improve participants' ability to respond appropriately to comments from others.
2. To improve participants' ability to distinguish between appropriate and inappropriate responses.

**Program Description:**
**Preparation:**
The leader should prepare cassette tape with recorded statements at intervals, such as:

- "You're so stupid!"
- "You're not my friend."
- "You can't come with us."
- "Thanks for the nice gift."
- "Could you help me with this problem?"

**Introduction:**
The purpose of this activity is to provide participants with the opportunity to express appropriate statements and apply these to daily situations within their personal lives.

**Activity Description:**
The leader states the goals and the purpose of the activity. Participants will listen to the prerecorded statements on the tape and write an appropriate response to each statement. The leader should instruct participants that they must write down their responses individually first and then they will have the opportunity to share with the group.

The prerecorded tape will be played to the participants and then they will be given a chance to respond appropriately. After each participant has been given the chance to respond to the statements, a discussion will take place about how responses can either be appropriate or inappropriate and how it feels when peers speak appropriately or inappropriately to one another.

All participants will have the opportunity to discuss any of the situations in which they are interested.

The leader should restate the goals and purpose of the activity and let the participants comment about what they learned.

**Debriefing Questions/Closure:**
1. How can you tell the difference between an appropriate response and an inappropriate response?
2. What actions should you take when your first reaction is an inappropriate response?
3. How do appropriate responses relate to maturity levels?

**Leadership Considerations:**
1. The leader should make statements relate to needs of the group.
2. The leader should be prepared if participants make an inappropriate response during the activity.

**Variations:**
1. The participants may create their own statement topics.
2. The participants may draw statements out of a hat.

**Creator:** Monika Ressel, Illinois State University, Normal, Illinois.

# My Friendship Windsock

**Space Requirements:** Classroom or activity room

**Equipment/Resource Requirements:** Plastic circles (with middle cut out), different colored cray paper, scissors, nylon string

**Group Size:** Small group

**Program Goals:**
1. To improve participants' ability to identify personal characteristics of being a friend.
2. To improve participants' ability to receive feedback from others.

**Program Description:**
**Preparation:**
The leader should gather materials and make a sample windsock for demonstration purposes.

**Introduction:**
The purpose of this activity is to improve the participants' ability to identify personal characteristics of being a friend and receiving feedback from peers.

**Activity Description:**
The leader begins by stating the goals and the purpose of the activity. The leader should explain that all participants are responsible for being honest about themselves. He or she should describe the different characteristics of friendship that will be represented (see examples). The leader will distribute plastic circles and cray paper strips. The participants will then build their windsocks using colors that represent their personal friendship characteristics using the following colors:

- blue—funny,
- green—understanding,
- yellow—good listener,
- white—quiet,
- red—impatient,
- black—patient,
- pink—happy, and
- orange—loud.

After building their friendship windsocks, all participants will have the opportunity to describe why they chose the colors they did. Other participants should give feedback about their reactions, agreement or disagreement.

The leader should restate the goals and the purpose of the activity and let the participants comment about what they learned.

Participants should be allowed to hang their windsocks in their rooms or outside near a window.

**Debriefing Questions/Closure:**
1. What three characteristics describe you best?
2. What three characteristics do you look for in a friend?
3. How are your characteristics similar to others in the group?
4. How are your characteristics different from others in the group?
5. What characteristics do you need to improve?
6. What did you learn by listening to feedback from other people?

**Leadership Considerations:**
1. Participants should know each other reasonably well.
2. The leader should allow ample time for discussion and feedback.

**Variation:**
Other materials may be used to build the windsocks.

**Creator:** Monika Ressel, Illinois State University, Normal, Illinois.

# The Mouse, the Monster, and Me

**Space Requirements:** Classroom or activity room

**Equipment/Resource Requirements:** Accompanying work sheet, pencils, area for participants to role-play

**Group Size:** Small group

**Program Goals:**
1. To improve participants' ability to identify passive, aggressive, and assertive behaviors.
2. To improve participants' ability to respond assertively to situations.
3. To improve participants' understanding that they can make choices regarding their individual behavior.

**Program Description:**
**Preparation:**
The leader should make one work sheet per participant.

**Introduction:**
The purpose of this activity is to distinguish between passive, aggressive, and assertive behaviors; develop assertive responses; and to understand each response is a choice.

**Activity Description:**
The leader will state the goals and the purpose of the activity. The group will discuss the differences between passive, assertive, and aggressive behaviors. The leader should explain and distribute the work sheet exercise and pencils. With assistance, the participants will write down situations in which they have been mice (passive), monsters (aggressive), and themselves (assertive).

After the participants have completed the work sheets, they will be given the opportunity to role-play their individual situations, and their peers will guess the situation. The leader will give the participants the opportunity to discuss how they can limit being mice and monsters, and maximize being themselves (assertive).

The leader should restate the goals and purpose of the activity and let the participants comment about what they learned.

**Debriefing Questions/Closure:**
1. What are some characteristics of being passive? What are some characteristics of being aggressive? What are some characteristics of being assertive?
2. What are the difficulties with being passive? What are the difficulties with being aggressive? What are the difficulties with being assertive?
3. What are the advantages to being assertive?
4. What do you need to do to become more assertive (and less passive or less aggressive)?
5. Name a situation coming up in the next week where you can practice your assertiveness skills.

**Leadership Considerations:**
1. The leader should know the differences between the three types of behaviors.
2. The leader should allow ample time for discussion.

**Variation:**
The leader could create scenarios for the participants to role-play.

**Creator:** Monika Ressel, Illinois State University, Normal, Illinois.

# The Mouse, the Monster, and Me

### The Mouse

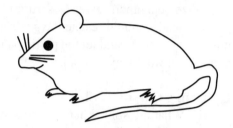

### The Monster

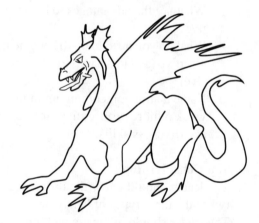

### Me!

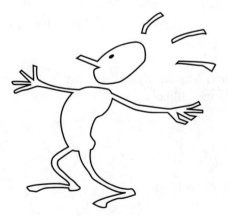

# Pass the Ketchup, Please

**Space Requirements:** Classroom or activity room

**Equipment/Resource Requirements:** Facility dining room or cafeteria, flatware, napkins, various food items, chart of table manners

**Group Size:** Small group

**Program Goal:**
To improve participants' knowledge and utilization of table manners and etiquette.

**Program Description:**
**Preparation:**
The leader should gather supplies. He or she could create a chart of table manners.

**Introduction:**
The purpose of this activity is to assist participants in acquiring, improving, and utilizing basic table manners.

**Activity Description:**
The leader should begin by stating the purpose and goal of this activity. This session should take place at the normal lunch or dinner hour and in the facility dining room or cafeteria. For each manner the leader will discuss and model expected behaviors. The participants should imitate the leader's behaviors. The leader and participants should practice manners prior to getting food.

*Manners:*
- Place napkin, unfolded, on lap.
- Avoid loud or sudden outbursts (in public).
- Correct use of utensils—forks for solid foods, knives only for spreading and cutting, and spoons for liquid foods and desserts.
- Place knife on edge of plate after using (do not hold knife while eating).
- Do not speak with food in mouth.
- Chew food with mouth closed.
- Avoid reaching for items on table; instead ask person closest to item to pass the item (e.g., "Please pass the salt").
- Body position—sit up straight, no elbows on table while eating.
- Avoid slurping soups and beverages.
- Do not bring mouth to food, bring food to mouth (e.g., do not bend head way down to the plate).

*Note:* The leader should use his or her discretion on the manners; some clients may not be physically able to do some of the required behaviors. The leader should ask these clients to do their best.

The leader should ask the participants if they have any questions. The leader should ask if they feel comfortable with the skills. If not, the participants should find out why and try to overcome resistance (many inappropriate table manners are habits and will be hard to break—do not get discouraged).

The participants should get their food. During the meal, the leader should cue the participants to correct behaviors by modeling skills in an exaggerated way. The leader should use verbal instruction for correction. The leader should be direct and clear, but not embarrass or shame the participant. He or she should reinforce correct behaviors.

After finishing the meal, the participants should clear the table and discuss the session.

**Debriefing Questions/Closure:**
1. What skills (manners) were you comfortable using? What skills (manners) were you uncomfortable using?
2. What skills, if any, do you feel are unnecessary? Why?

3. What skills were easy to remember? What skills were difficult to remember?
4. Table manners make eating a more pleasant experience. What skill will you work hardest to improve on?

**Leadership Considerations:**
1. The leader must demonstrate appropriate table manners.

2. The leader should allow participants to practice and self-correct.

**Variation:**
Mirrors may be placed in front of participants so they can monitor their own behavior.

**Creator:** Susan Osborn, Illinois State University, Normal, Illinois.

# Are You Passive, Aggressive, or Assertive?

**Space Requirements:** Classroom or activity room

**Equipment/Resource Requirements:** Passive, aggressive, and assertive cards (one set per participant), scenarios which relate to the issues being faced by specific population

**Group Size:** Small group

**Program Goals:**
1. To increase participants' knowledge of the differences between passivity, aggressiveness, and assertiveness.
2. To improve participants' ability to identify characteristics related to assertiveness.
3. To increase participants' ability to follow directions and stay on task.

**Program Description:**
**Preparation:**
Prior to the activity, the leader should have all materials prepared, including note cards and scenarios. The leader should create scenarios appropriate to the participants.

**Introduction:**
The purpose of this activity is to increase the participants' knowledge of and their ability to identify characteristics related to assertiveness.

**Activity Description:**
The leader should introduce the activity to the group by explaining that it will deal with the differences between being assertive and being passive or aggressive. The leader will begin the activity by leading a discussion which identifies and defines passive behaviors, aggressive behaviors, and assertive behaviors. The leader should have examples of each prepared to aid in the explanation of the three terms.

Following the discussion, the leader will explain that a list of situations that relate to each of the three behaviors has been prepared and will be read to the group. Additionally, the leader will explain that they will each receive three note cards. Once note cards are distributed, the leader should ensure that each of the participants has one card stating *passive,* one card stating *aggressive,* and one card stating *assertive.*

The leader should explain to the group that each scenario will involve an interaction between two or more people. The job of the participant is to identify the behaviors of each character involved in the scenario. Participants are to label the behaviors of the named individual from the scenario as being passive, aggressive, or assertive. Each of the participants will do this individually.

An example may include:

*Scenario:* Georgene arrived at Tots in Trouble to meet with her supervisor to discuss the activities she has implemented with the 9- to 11-year-old girls. Georgene is very frustrated with the behaviors the girls exhibit. Georgene's supervisor, Trisha, asks Georgene, "How did group go last week?" Georgene replies angrily, "The group went awful. If things don't shape up around here, I refuse to continue implementing groups with these girls."

The leader would then ask the participant to hold up the card that identifies Georgene's behavior. In this case, Georgene's behavior would be labeled as aggressive.

The leader should have 15 to 20 scenarios prepared for the group session. Scenarios should include a variety of all three behaviors—passive, aggressive, and assertive.

After each scenario, the group should discuss the correct answer (behavior), and brainstorm how passive and aggressive behaviors can be changed to be more assertive. When all of the scenarios have been discussed or time runs out, the leader will discuss the following debriefing questions as a group.

**Debriefing Questions/Closure:**

1. Now that we have discussed the scenarios, please create your own definition of passive, aggressive, and assertive behaviors, and share them with the group.
2. Name some situations in your life where someone has been passive, aggressive, and/or assertive.
3. How do you feel and/or respond when someone acts passively toward you? How do you feel and/or respond when someone acts aggressively toward you? How do you feel and/or respond when someone acts assertively toward you?
4. How do you feel when you act passively towards others? How do you feel when you act aggressively towards others? How do you feel when you act assertively towards others?
5. Identify methods you can implement to assist you in becoming more assertive.

**Leadership Considerations:**

1. The leader should ensure that all participants understand the definitions of each behavior before beginning the scenario exercise.
2. The leader should ensure all participants have responded before giving the correct answer to each scenario.

**Variations:**

1. Group members could act out scenarios and other individuals could identify behaviors.
2. Individuals could provide real-life situations they encountered and identify how they behaved or reacted in those situations.
3. The leader could create an assertiveness game where participants are placed on teams and each time a team identifies a correct behavior a point is awarded.

**Creator:** Theresa M. Connolly, CTRS, Illinois State University, Normal, Illinois.

# Social Skittles

**Space Requirements:** Classroom or activity room

**Equipment/Resource Requirements:** Skittles candy, construction paper, black marker, small plastic bags

**Group Size:** Small group

**Program Goals:**
1. To improve participants' ability to verbalize positive characteristics of themselves.
2. To improve participants' ability to verbalize positive characteristics of other group members.

**Program Description:**
**Preparation:**
The leader should gather materials and put a variety of colored Skittles in plastic bags, one bag for each group member.

**Introduction:**
The purpose of this activity is to improve participants' ability to verbalize positive characteristics about themselves and others.

**Activity Description:**
The leader begins by stating the goals and the purpose of the activity. The group forms a circle sitting at the same level. The leader must then distribute the bags of candy to the participants and choose one participant to start. For each color of Skittles, the participant is to follow the directions:

- Green—Something nice about the person to your left.
- Yellow—Something you like about yourself.
- Purple—Favorite thing to do with friends.

- Orange—Something that you would like to become better at.
- Red—Something nice about the person to your right.

The leader should describe to the participants that for every color of candy they must say something, following what each color means. The leader should encourage the participants to use positive statements.

Charts should be placed around the room with the statements written on the colors coinciding with the statements. Each person in the group takes a turn. If the participant can't think of anything positive to say, the Skittle is given to the leader. After everyone is finished, the Skittles can be eaten by the participants.

The leader should restate the goals and purpose of the activity and let the participants comment about what they learned.

**Debriefing Questions/Closure:**
1. How easy or difficult was it to come up with positive statements?
2. Why is it important to recognize positive characteristics in yourself and others?
3. What can you do to be more positive every day?

**Leadership Considerations:**
1. The leader will make sure that participants are generating ideas through the other group members' responses. The leader will make sure each member is given enough time to fully answer the question and use positive statements.
2. The leader should make sure that the participants wait their turns and respect the answers of all of the other group members.

**Variation:**
Once each group member receives a turn and everyone has followed directions appropriately, the participants could switch seating arrangements to allow the questions to be answered differently.

**Creator:** Monika Ressel, Illinois State University, Normal, Illinois.

# Index of Contributors

# Other Books From Venture Publishing, Inc.

*The A•B•Cs of Behavior Change: Skills for Working With Behavior Problems in Nursing Homes*
    by Margaret D. Cohn, Michael A. Smyer, and Ann L. Horgas

*Activity Experiences and Programming Within Long-Term Care*
    by Ted Tedrick and Elaine R. Green

*The Activity Gourmet*
    by Peggy Powers

*Advanced Concepts for Geriatric Nursing Assistants*
    by Carolyn A. McDonald

*Adventure Education*
    edited by John C. Miles and Simon Priest

*Aerobics of the Mind: Keeping the Mind Active in Aging—A New Perspective on Programming for Older Adults*
    by Marge Engelman

*Assessment: The Cornerstone of Activity Programs*
    by Ruth Perschbacher

*Behavior Modification in Therapeutic Recreation: An Introductory Manual*
    by John Datillo and William D. Murphy

*Benefits of Leisure*
    edited by B. L. Driver, Perry J. Brown, and George L. Peterson

*Benefits of Recreation Research Update*
    by Judy M. Sefton and W. Kerry Mummery

*Beyond Bingo: Innovative Programs for the New Senior*
    by Sal Arrigo, Jr., Ann Lewis, and Hank Mattimore

*Beyond Bingo 2: More Innovative Programs for the New Senior*
    by Sal Arrigo, Jr.

*Both Gains and Gaps: Feminist Perspectives on Women's Leisure*
    by Karla Henderson, M. Deborah Bialeschki, Susan M. Shaw, and Valeria J. Freysinger

*Dimensions of Choice: A Qualitative Approach to Recreation, Parks, and Leisure Research*
    by Karla A. Henderson

*Effective Management in Therapeutic Recreation Service*
    by Gerald S. O'Morrow and Marcia Jean Carter

*Evaluating Leisure Services: Making Enlightened Decisions*
    by Karla A. Henderson with M. Deborah Bialeschki

*Everything From A to Y: The Zest Is up to You! Older Adult Activities for Every Day of the Year*
    by Nancy R. Cheshire and Martha L. Kenney

*The Evolution of Leisure: Historical and Philosophical Perspectives (Second Printing)*
    by Thomas Goodale and Geoffrey Godbey

*Experience Marketing: Strategies for the New Millennium*
    by Ellen L. O'Sullivan and Kathy J. Spangler

*File o' Fun: A Recreation Planner for Games & Activities—Third Edition*
    by Jane Harris Ericson and Diane Ruth Albright

*The Game Finder—A Leader's Guide to Great Activities*
    by Annette C. Moore

*Getting People Involved in Life and Activities: Effective Motivating Techniques*
    by Jeanne Adams

*Great Special Events and Activities*
    by Annie Morton, Angie Prosser, and Sue Spangler

*Inclusive Leisure Services: Responding to the Rights of People With Disabilities*
    by John Dattilo

*Internships in Recreation and Leisure Services: A Practical Guide for Students (Second Edition)*
    by Edward E. Seagle, Jr., Ralph W. Smith, and Lola M. Dalton

*Interpretation of Cultural and Natural Resources*
    by Douglas M. Knudson, Ted T. Cable, and Larry Beck

*Introduction to Leisure Services—7th Edition*
    by H. Douglas Sessoms and Karla A. Henderson

*Leadership and Administration of Outdoor Pursuits, Second Edition*
    by Phyllis Ford and James Blanchard
*Leadership in Leisure Services: Making a Difference*
    by Debra J. Jordan
*Leisure and Leisure Services in the 21st Century*
    by Geoffrey Godbey
*The Leisure Diagnostic Battery: Users Manual and Sample Forms*
    by Peter A. Witt and Gary Ellis
*Leisure Education: A Manual of Activities and Resources*
    by Norma J. Stumbo and Steven R. Thompson
*Leisure Education II: More Activities and Resources*
    by Norma J. Stumbo
*Leisure Education III: More Goal-Oriented Activities*
    by Norma J. Stumbo
*Leisure Education IV: Activities for Individuals With Substance Addictions*
    by Norma J. Stumbo
*Leisure Education Program Planning: A Systematic Approach—Second Edition*
    by John Dattilo
*Leisure in Your Life: An Exploration—Fifth Edition*
    by Geoffrey Godbey
*Leisure Services in Canada: An Introduction*
    by Mark S. Searle and Russell E. Brayley
*Leisure Studies: Prospects for the Twenty-First Century*
    edited by Edgar L. Jackson and Thomas L. Burton
*The Lifestory Re-Play Circle: A Manual of Activities and Techniques*
    by Rosilyn Wilder
*Marketing for Parks, Recreation, and Leisure*
    by Ellen L. O'Sullivan
*Models of Change in Municipal Parks and Recreation: A Book of Innovative Case Studies*
    edited by Mark E. Havitz
*More Than a Game: A New Focus on Senior Activity Services*
    by Brenda Corbett
*Nature and the Human Spirit: Toward an Expanded Land Management Ethic*
    edited by B. L. Driver, Daniel Dustin, Tony Baltic, Gary Elsner, and George Peterson

*Outdoor Recreation Management: Theory and Application, Third Edition*
    by Alan Jubenville and Ben Twight
*Planning Parks for People, Second Edition*
    by John Hultsman, Richard L. Cottrell, and Wendy Z. Hultsman
*The Process of Recreation Programming Theory and Technique, Third Edition*
    by Patricia Farrell and Herberta M. Lundegren
*Programming for Parks, Recreation, and Leisure Services: A Servant Leadership Approach*
    by Donald G. DeGraaf, Debra J. Jordan, and Kathy H. DeGraaf
*Protocols for Recreation Therapy Programs*
    edited by Jill Kelland, along with the Recreation Therapy Staff at Alberta Hospital Edmonton
*Quality Management: Applications for Therapeutic Recreation*
    edited by Bob Riley
*A Recovery Workbook: The Road Back From Substance Abuse*
    by April K. Neal and Michael J. Taleff
*Recreation and Leisure: Issues in an Era of Change, Third Edition*
    edited by Thomas Goodale and Peter A. Witt
*Recreation Economic Decisions: Comparing Benefits and Costs (Second Edition)*
    by John B. Loomis and Richard G. Walsh
*Recreation Programming and Activities for Older Adults*
    by Jerold E. Elliott and Judith A. Sorg-Elliott
*Recreation Programs That Work for At-Risk Youth: The Challenge of Shaping the Future*
    by Peter A. Witt and John L. Crompton
*Reference Manual for Writing Rehabilitation Therapy Treatment Plans*
    by Penny Hogberg and Mary Johnson
*Research in Therapeutic Recreation: Concepts and Methods*
    edited by Marjorie J. Malkin and Christine Z. Howe
*Simple Expressions: Creative and Therapeutic Arts for the Elderly in Long-Term Care Facilities*
    by Vicki Parsons
*A Social History of Leisure Since 1600*
    by Gary Cross
*A Social Psychology of Leisure*
    by Roger C. Mannell and Douglas A. Kleiber

Venture Publishing, Inc.
1999 Cato Avenue
State College, PA 16801

Phone: (814) 234-4561; Fax: (814) 234-1651